# Rheumatology
# Board Review

# Rheumatology Board Review

Editor

## Karen Law, MD

Assistant Professor of Medicine
Division of Rheumatology
Emory University School of Medicine
Atlanta, GA, USA

Associate Editor

## Aliza Lipson, MD

Assistant Professor of Medicine
Division of Rheumatology
Emory University School of Medicine
Atlanta, GA, USA

WILEY Blackwell

*Library of Congress Cataloging-in-Publication Data*
Rheumatology board review / editor, Karen Law ; associate editor, Aliza Lipson.
       p. ; cm.
    Includes bibliographical references and index.
    ISBN 978-1-118-12791-9 (pbk. : alk. paper) – ISBN 978-1-118-47584-3 (ePub) –
ISBN 978-1-118-47594-2 (ePdf) – ISBN 978-1-118-47596-6 (eMobi) – ISBN 978-1-118-47597-3
    I. Law, Karen, editor of compilation.   II. Lipson, Aliza, editor of compilation.
    [DNLM: 1. Rheumatic Diseases–Outlines.   2. Rheumatology–Outlines.   WE 18.2]
    RC927
    616.7′230076–dc23
                                            2013026486

Cover image: Top image – iStock file #22909211 © zhongguo. Middle image – iStock file #2291786 © Dominik Pabis. Bottom image – iStock file #16004426 © GeorgHanf.
Cover design by Matt Kuhns

# Contents

# List of Contributors

**Sheila Angeles-Han, MD, MSc**

Assistant Professor of Pediatrics and
Ophthalmology
Division of Pediatric Rheumatology
Emory University School of Medicine
Children's Healthcare of Atlanta
Atlanta, GA, USA

**Schartess Culpepper-Pace, MD**

Rheumatology and Internal Medicine
Chen Medical Centers
Miami, FL, USA

**Cristina Drenkard, MD, PhD**

Assistant Professor of Medicine
Division of Rheumatology
Emory University School of Medicine
Atlanta, GA, USA

**Robin Geletka, MD**

Rheumatology Medical Science Liaison
Actelion Pharmaceuticals Ltd
San Francisco, CA, USA

**Arezou Khosroshahi, MD**

Assistant Professor of Medicine
Division of Rheumatology
Emory University School of Medicine
Atlanta, GA, USA

**Karen Law, MD**

Assistant Professor of Medicine
Division of Rheumatology
Emory University School of Medicine
Atlanta, GA, USA

**S. Sam Lim, MD, MPH**

Associate Professor of Medicine
Clinical Director, Division of Rheumatology
Emory University School of Medicine
Atlanta, GA, USA

**Aliza Lipson, MD**

Assistant Professor of Medicine
Division of Rheumatology
Emory University School of Medicine
Atlanta, GA, USA

**Courtney McCracken, PhD**

Department of Pediatrics
Emory University School of Medicine
Atlanta, GA, USA

**Laura Paxton, MD**

Clinical Instructor of Medicine
Division of Rheumatology
Atlanta Veterans Affairs Medical Center;
Emory University School of Medicine
Atlanta, GA, USA

**John Payan, MD, MPA**

Section Chief of Musculoskeletal Imaging
Atlanta Veterans Affairs Medical Center;
Assistant Professor of Radiology
Emory University School of Medicine
Atlanta, GA, USA

**Sampath Prahalad, MD, MS**

Marcus Professor of Pediatric Rheumatology
Chief, Division of Pediatric Rheumatology
Associate Professor of Pediatrics and Human
Genetics
Emory University School of Medicine
Children's Healthcare of Atlanta
Atlanta, GA, USA

**Gnanesh Patel, MD**

Fellow in Rheumatology
Emory University School of Medicine
Atlanta, GA, USA

**Kelly A. Rouster-Stevens, MD, MS**

Assistant Professor of Pediatrics
Division of Pediatric Rheumatology
Emory University School of Medicine
Children's Healthcare of Atlanta
Atlanta, GA, USA

**Iñaki Sanz, MD**

Mason I. Lowance Professor of Medicine and
Pediatrics
Chief, Division of Rheumatology
Director, Lowance Center for Human
Immunology
Emory University School of Medicine
Atlanta, GA, USA

**Athan Tiliakos, DO**

Assistant Professor of Medicine
Division of Rheumatology
Emory University School of Medicine
Atlanta, GA, USA

**Larry Vogler, MD**

Associate Professor of Pediatrics
Division of Pediatric Rheumatology
Emory University School of Medicine
Children's Healthcare of Atlanta
Atlanta, GA, USA

# Preface

*Rheumatology Board Review* is offered as an up-to-date, concise review of the rheumatic diseases, with an emphasis on recent advances in the field, including immune-modulating and biologic medications, new classification criteria, pediatric topics, and new paradigms of treatment. Each chapter employs an outline format designed to efficiently convey a maximum amount of material, accented by simple figures, radiographs, and tables to enhance understanding.

This book is dedicated to health professionals at all levels of training who share an interest in our ever-evolving, fascinating field of rheumatology. We hope this book contributes to a deeper understanding of topics in the rheumatic diseases and a lifelong interest in rheumatology.

Karen Law
Aliza Lipson

# CHAPTER 1

# Non-inflammatory joint and soft tissue disorders

**Laura Paxton[1,3], Schartess Culpepper-Pace[2], Karen Law[3]**

[1]Atlanta Veterans Affairs Medical Center, Atlanta, GA, USA
[2]Rheumatology and Internal Medicine, Chen Medical Centers, Miami, FL, USA
[3]Emory University School of Medicine, Atlanta, GA, USA

## Introduction

Rheumatologists often manage non-inflammatory arthritides and associated soft tissue disorders, including osteoarthritis, carpal tunnel syndrome, and gout. The diagnosis of these conditions as well as recent innovations in treatment will be reviewed here.

## Carpal tunnel syndrome

### Epidemiology
- One of the most common and frequently diagnosed entrapment neuropathies
  - Accounts for up to 90% of entrapment neuropathies
  - Prevalence in the US population up to 5% of the general population
    - Estimated lifetime risk of 10%
    - Females affected more frequently than men
    - Peak age range 40–60 years

---

*Rheumatology Board Review*, First Edition. Edited by Karen Law and Aliza Lipson.
© 2014 John Wiley & Sons, Inc. Published 2014 by John Wiley & Sons, Inc.

○ Risk factors include prolonged wrist flexion or extension, repeated use of flexor muscles, and exposure to vibration
  ▪ Systemic medical conditions i.e. diabetes, hypothyroidism, obesity, pregnancy, vitamin toxicity or deficiency can predispose
  ▪ Many cases remain idiopathic

## Pathology

• Median nerve entrapment is caused by chronic pressure at the level of the carpal tunnel
• Compression of the median nerve is secondary to surrounding structures: **carpal bones, flexor tendons**, and the fibrous **transverse carpal ligament** leading to median nerve dysfunction
  ○ Carpal tunnel anatomy (Figure 1.1)
    ▪ Superiorly: transverse carpal ligament
    ▪ Posteriorly: carpal bones
    ▪ Nine flexor tendons: (four) flexor digitorum profundus, (four) flexor digitorum superficialis, flexor pollicis
    ▪ Median nerve
• Repetitive compressive injury to the median nerve leads to demyelination
  ○ Blood flow may also be interrupted, altering the blood–nerve barrier

## Clinical presentation

• Symptoms may include tingling and numbness, in the distribution of the median nerve (**first three fingers and radial aspect of the fourth finger**); pain involving the entire hand, decreased grip strength, and reduced dexterity

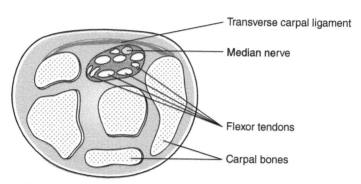

**Figure 1.1** Components of the carpal tunnel (Color plate 1.1).

- Feet – first metatarsophalangeal (MTP), subtalar joint
- Knee
- Hip
- Spine
- Rarely affects elbow, wrist, ankle – look for history of trauma, congenital abnormality, systemic or crystalline disease

## Definition
- OA can be defined pathologically, radiographically, or clinically
- Radiographic OA has long been considered the reference standard for epidemiology
  - **Not all subjects with radiographic OA are symptomatic and not all with symptoms have radiographic OA**

## Risk factors
- Age – the strongest risk factor, most commonly age >40 years
- Females
- Obesity – the strongest **modifiable** risk factor
- Previous injury
- Family history (genetic predisposition)
- Joint malalignment (mechanical factors)

## Pathogenesis
- Caused by an interplay of multiple factors – joint integrity, genetics, local inflammation, mechanical forces, cellular and biochemical processes
- Abnormal remodeling of joint tissues is driven by a host of inflammatory mediators within the joint
- OA pathogenesis is now thought of as an **active response to injury** rather than a degenerative process
  - Degradation of matrix and articular cartilage
    - Chondrocytes become "activated" and increase production of matrix proteins and matrix-degrading enzymes during inadequate repair response
      - → Aggrecanases, collagenases, serine and cysteine proteinases, matrix metalloproteinase (MMP)-3, MMP-13, ADAMTS-5 are all reported to play a role
  - Thickening of the subchondral bone
    - Bone remodeling may be initiated at sites of local bone damage resulting from excessive repetitive loading
  - Formation of osteophytes
    - At joint margins and entheseal sites – new bone is added by endochondral ossification, leading to osteophyte formation

○ Variable degrees of inflammation of the synovium
   ▪ Synovial infiltrates have been identified in many OA patients, though lower in grade than in rheumatoid arthritis (RA)
   ▪ Prevalence of synovitis increases with advancing age
   ▪ **Interleukin (IL)-1 beta** and **tumor necrosis factor (TNF) alpha** suppress matrix synthesis and promote cartilage catabolism, **IL-17** induces chemokine production by synovial fibroblasts and chondrocytes
○ Degeneration of ligaments, menisci in the knee, and hypertrophy of the joint capsule, as any meniscal or ligamentous injury predisposes to the development of OA

## Symptoms
- Hand
  ○ Pain on usage
  ○ Mild morning or inactivity stiffness, usually lasting <30 minutes
  ○ Characteristic sites – DIPs, PIPs, base of the thumb
- Knee and hip
  ○ Usage-related pain
  ○ Often worse toward the end of the day
  ○ Pain relieved, usually incompletely, with rest
  ○ Mild morning or inactivity stiffness (gelling)
  ○ Advanced OA – may have rest or night pain
  ○ OA symptoms are often episodic or variable in severity and slow to change

## Physical examination
- Hand
  ○ Heberden's (DIPs) and Bouchard's (PIPs) nodes
  ○ Squared appearance to the first CMC is classic
- Feet
  ○ First MTP involvement may result in hallux valgus or hallux rigidus
- Knees
  ○ Tenderness to palpation of joint
  ○ Crepitus
  ○ Joint effusion
    ▪ Synovial fluid in OA typically exhibits
      → Normal viscosity
      → Mild pleocytosis (WBC <2000/mm$^3$)
  ○ Osteophytes – may have palpable bony enlargements at periphery of joint
  ○ Restricted movement and range of motion

- Hip
  - Hip pain worsened with internal or external rotation
  - Anterior and inguinal pain generally indicative of true hip joint involvement
  - Check both hips, as ~20% have bilateral OA
  - Full exam should also include evaluation for referred pain sources
    - Trochanteric bursitis
    - Lumbosacral spine
    - Knee pathology

## Osteoarthritis treatment

Management is primarily symptomatic, as no treatments have been shown to slow or reverse joint damage. Patient education regarding the natural history of the disease is critical. Non-pharmacologic treatments must be balanced with judicious use of pharmacologic treatments.

### Non-pharmacologic treatments
- Instruction on joint protection techniques
- Thermal modalities – paraffin wax treatments, heat packs, and heating pads
- Strong recommendation for **weight loss** in patients with hip or knee OA
- Exercise – cardiovascular and/or resistance land-based exercise, aquatic exercise, and manual therapy (physical/occupational therapy) in combination with supervised exercise have all been helpful
- Participation in self-management programs and psychosocial interventions (diet, exercise instruction) can offer significant benefit
- Tai chi programs have been reported to be beneficial in small studies
- Assistive devices, orthotics, and splinting as needed:
  - Splints for trapeziometacarpal joint OA
  - Medially wedged insoles for lateral compartment knee OA
  - Laterally wedged subtalar strapped insoles for medial compartment knee OA
  - Medially directed patellar taping for knee OA

### Pharmacologic therapy
- Acetaminophen
- Topical capsaicin – efficacy is controversial, but some advocate for its use as adjunctive treatment

- Topical non-steroidal anti-inflammatory drugs (NSAIDs), e.g. topical diclofenac, is a safe option especially if age >75 years
- Oral NSAIDs, including non-selective and selective (cyclo-oxygenase (COX)-2 inhibitors) (Table 1.1)
  - Monitor for gastrointestinal (GI) and cardiac adverse effects (GI bleeding, abdominal pain, MI, worsening CHF)
  - Avoid in chronic kidney disease
  - COX-2 selective inhibitors are associated with increased cardiovascular risk and should be avoided in patients with cardiovascular risk factors
- Tramadol can also play a role in pain relief, especially in patients for whom NSAIDs or acetaminophen are contraindicated
- Intra-articular injection of long-acting corticosteroid can be effective for painful flares of OA, especially in trapeziometacarpal joint OA and knee OA

### Intra-articular viscosupplementation
- Multiple brands available (Table 1.2)
  - Currently only FDA-approved for knee osteoarthritis
  - Few head-to-head comparisons and generally small studies
- Mechanism
  - Hyaluronic acid (HA) is a constitutive component of the matrix cartilage
    - Plays a key role in maintenance of joint homeostasis
    - Biologically active component secreted by chondrocytes that protects cartilage from degradation by interacting with MMPs and pain mediators
    - In OA, concentration and molecular weight of HA is reduced

**Table 1.1** Use of NSAIDs in high-risk populations.

| Clinical scenario | Recommended regimen |
|---|---|
| History of GI bleed, but none within the past year | Non-selective NSAID or COX-2 inhibitor + proton-pump inhibitor |
| History of GI bleed within the past year | COX-2 inhibitor + proton-pump inhibitor |
| Patient taking low-dose aspirin for cardioprotection | Non-selective NSAID other than ibuprofen* + proton-pump inhibitor |

*The FDA warns against ibuprofen and low-dose aspirin used in combination, due to a pharmacodynamic interaction causing a decreased cardiprotective effect

**Table 1.2** Comparison of viscosupplementation products.

| Product | Dosing | Molecular weight (in M Daltons) |
| --- | --- | --- |
| Hyalgan (sodium hyaluronate) | Once weekly for 3–5 weeks | 0.5–0.73 |
| Supartz (sodium hyaluronate) | Once weekly for 3–5 weeks | 0.6–1.1 |
| Orthovisc (high molecular weight hyaluronan) | Once weekly for 3–4 weeks | 1.0–2.9 |
| Euflexxa (1% sodium hyaluronate) | Once weekly for 3 weeks | 2.4–3.6 |
| Synvisc (hylan G-F 20) | Once weekly for 3 weeks | 6 |
| Synvisc-One (hylan G-F 20) | Once | 6 |

- ○ Exact mechanism not understood
- ○ Proposed mechanism
  - ▪ Biomechanical – improves synovial fluid viscoelasticity, increases joint lubrication, coats articular cartilage surface
  - ▪ Analgesic – reduces pain eliciting nerve activity, reduces prostaglandin- or bradykinin-induced pain
  - ▪ Anti-inflammatory – reduces levels of inflammatory mediators, decreases leukocyte chemotaxis
  - ▪ Antioxidant
  - ▪ Chondroprotective – stimulation of endogenous HA and extra matrix component synthesis, protects against chondrocyte apoptosis, inhibits cartilage degradation
- • Side effects
  - ○ Generally well tolerated, most side effects related to injection site reactions
  - ○ Rare **pseudosepsis reactions**, especially with high molecular weight HA
    - ▪ Patients present with acute joint swelling, pain, and warmth
    - ▪ Care must be taken to distinguish this syndrome from true septic joint
- • Clinical use
  - ○ Used in knee OA patients who fail non-pharmacologic treatments, acetaminophen, NSAIDs, and intra-articular steroids
  - ○ Studies have shown improvement in pain scores with viscosupplementation, however:
    - ▪ Appropriate patient selection is not well defined
    - ▪ Many studies do not control for concomitant pharmacologic therapy
    - ▪ Double-blind, placebo-controlled trials report a large placebo effect

○ Campbell et al. in 2007 reviewed six systematic reviews on viscosupplementation
  ▪ Three reviews showed viscosupplementation more effective than placebo
  ▪ Three reviews suggested no benefit
○ Rutjes et al. in 2012 systematic review and meta-analysis concluded that viscosupplementation is associated with a small and clinically irrelevant benefit and an increased risk for serious adverse events
○ Viscosupplementation is not recommended for OA of the hip due to lack of data

### Glucosamine and chondroitin sulfate

• Both are labeled as supplements in the United States and are therefore do not need to be approved by the FDA before they are marketed; therefore variations in dosage among the marketed supplements exist, making comparisons difficult
• The GAIT trial for knee OA demonstrated that response to glucosamine and chondroitin alone or in combination were not different from placebo
  ○ A small subgroup analysis of patients with moderate-to-severe knee OA did show statistically significant improvement with combination therapy
  ○ 2-year follow up did not demonstrate clinically significant differences between the treatment groups
• Other studies have shown efficacy with these agents but were criticized for flaws, including failure to adhere to intention to treat, small numbers of patients, potential bias related to sponsorship of the study, and inadequate masking of the study agent
• As a result, recommendations from leading organizations differ:
  ○ American College of Rheumatology (ACR) 2012 statement recommends against the use of glucosamine and chondroitin
  ○ European League against Rheumatism (EULAR) recommendations include glucosamine and chondroitin as viable treatment option for knee OA
  ○ OARSI (Osteoarthritis Research Society International) recommends a trial for 6 months, followed by reassessment and discontinuation if ineffective at that time

### Surgery for osteoarthritis

• Joint replacement for the knee and hip should be considered in patients with radiographic evidence of OA along with chronic pain and disability

that is refractory to treatment with non-pharmacologic and pharmacologic interventions
• Surgical intervention should be performed before the development of
significant deformities, contractures, functional loss, or muscle atrophy
for optimal result

> Knee surgical options include arthroscopy, osteotomy, and total knee
> arthroplasty. The type of surgical procedure is dependent on the location
> and stage of OA, comorbidities, age and physical activity level, and the
> degree of patient symptoms.

○ Arthroscopic lavage and debridement
  ▪ Role in knee OA is controversial
  ▪ Lack of evidence to show significant benefit
○ Unloading osteotomy
  ▪ Can be used in young and active patients with unicompartmental
  OA
  ▪ Aim to unload damaged compartment and transfer weight by
  slightly overcorrecting into a valgus or varus axis
  ▪ Must have appropriate patient selection for satisfactory outcome
  ▪ Typically good results in the first few years, however, satisfaction
  decreases thereafter
○ Arthroplasty
  ▪ Unicompartmental knee arthroplasty
    → Indicated when OA involves only one compartment of the knee
    → Appropriate for younger patients with less severe disease
    → More rapid recovery
    → Provides preservation of bone stock, more normal knee kinemat-
    ics, greater physiologic function
    → Poorer long-term survival of prosthetic than total knee
    arthroplasty
  ▪ Total knee arthroplasty (TKA)
    → Indicated in advanced OA with more than one compartment
    involved
    → Durability of prosthetic components is approximately 15–20
    years, therefore it is typically avoided in patients <60 years old
    → Main complications – femoropatellar problems, loosening of
    components, infections, residual stiffness

Hip surgical options are less varied than knee surgical options. Hip resurfacing is an option for young, more active patients who have an interest in a bone-conserving replacement procedure. Total hip arthroplasty (THA) has excellent long-term results in the treatment of late, symptomatic OA. Complications for THA are similar to those for TKA.

## Secondary osteoarthritis

Secondary osteoarthritis is caused by previous injury or disease of the target joint, due to conditions that adversely alter the articular cartilage or subchondral bone. Conditions that predispose to the development of secondary OA include trauma, infections, prior surgery, mineral deposition, and autoimmune disorders. Several of these conditions will be discussed further in this section.

## Etiologies
- Metabolic
  - **Crystal-associated arthritis** (gout, pseudogout)
    - Both monosodium urate (MSU) and calcium-containing crystals (calcium pyrophosphate dihydrate [CPPD], basic calcium phosphate crystals) may contribute to inflammation in OA tissues through direct interactions with components of the innate immune system and the amplification of other inflammatory signals
    - Calcium-containing crystals are frequently found in tissues from patients with end-stage OA
  - **Ochronosis** (hereditary alkaptonuria)
    - A rare hereditary autosomal recessive disease characterized by a defect in the gene coding for homogentisate 1,2–dioxygenase leading to accumulation of homogentisic acid
    - Black pigment produced by oxidation and polymerization of homogentisic acid deposits in connective tissues and binds irreversibly to them, causing ochronosis
    - Clinical manifestations
      → Arthropathy causing degeneration of major joints and intervertebral discs
      → Can also affect skin and sclera
      → Patients tend to be asymptomatic until approximately 30 years of age, when sequelae of ochronosis becomes apparent

→ Ochronotic arthritis may begin in the late 30s with low back pain and stiffness; knee symptoms resemble typical osteoarthritis

→ Symptoms simulate degenerative joint disease – articular space narrowing, bone sclerosis, effusion

→ Cartilage tends to be more easily damaged, promoting rapid progression to end–stage disease

- Radiographic findings
  → Spine
    ○ Plain film and computed tomography (CT) scans of the spine show multilevel narrowing of intervertebral spaces, calcification, and vacuum phenomenon of intervertebral discs
  → Peripheral joints
    ○ Primarily affects weight-bearing joints (frequently knees, but also can involve hips, shoulders)
    ○ Joint space narrowing and subchondral sclerosis with cyst formation are apparent with minimal osteophytes
- Treatment is primarily symptomatic for early-stage disease, with many patients progressing to total joint replacement as end-stage joint disease develops

○ **Hemochromatosis**
- A relatively prevalent genetic disease characterized by tissue iron overload
- Most frequent mutation is the **homozygous C282Y gene mutation**
- Patients can develop life-threatening organ damage – liver cirrhosis, carcinoma, diabetes, and heart failure
- Other complications include arthropathy and osteoporosis; **pseudogout** is also commonly seen in patients with hemochromatosis
- Diagnosis
  → Clinical symptoms
    - Chronic weakness
    - Arthralgias/arthritis
    - Chondrocalcinosis
    - Bronze skin pigmentation
    - Unexplained liver disease or hepatomegaly
    - Type 1 diabetes
    - Early onset osteopenia/osteoporosis
    - Cardiac symptoms (rhythm disturbances, cardiac failure)
- Laboratory abnormalities
  → Plasma transferrin saturation and ferritin are increased
  → Must rule out increased ferritin from non-hemochromatosis causes – alcohol, inflammation, cell necrosis, dysmetabolic iron overload syndrome

- Joint manifestations
  - → Arthritis is common
    - ○ If present, symptoms often precede diagnosis by up to 9 years
    - ○ Two thirds of patients report joint symptoms as a major cause of impaired quality of life
    - ○ One third of hemochromatosis cases are revealed through the workup of isolated articular pain
  - → Symptoms can begin before 30 years of age in men but usually after menopause in women
  - → Joint location
    - ○ Classic joints involved – second and third metacarpophalangeals (MCPs)
      - Bony enlargement over second and third MCPs is common
    - ○ Other common joint involvement – wrists, PIPs, hips, knees, ankles
    - ○ Less frequent locations – shoulders, elbows, spine
  - → Can have either a monoarthritis or polyarthritis and pain crises
  - → Synovial fluid and laboratory studies may show either a degenerative or inflammatory profile
- Radiological manifestations:
  - → Most often seen in second and third MCPs
  - → Hook-shaped osteophytes of the MCPs is very characteristic with associated joint space narrowing
  - → Wrist and distal radioulnar joints are frequently affected
  - → Can sometimes lead to erosive arthritis which can mimic RA
  - → Chondrocalcinosis may also be seen, indicating concomitant CPPD
- Treatment:
  - → Iron removal by phlebotomy is often not helpful for joint symptoms
  - → No evidence based treatment to date
  - → NSAIDs and intra-articular glucocorticosteroids can be effective
  - → Treatment for pseudogout, if present, can also alleviate symptoms
- **Wilson's disease**
  - A rare autosomal recessive disorder characterized by release of free copper and accumulation of intracellular hepatic copper with subsequent hepatic and central nervous system abnormalities
  - Associated with **mutations of ATP7B gene**

- Peripheral joint manifestations – described in small open studies and case reports
  - → Often spontaneous or mechanical type arthralgias
  - → Patients report mono- or polyarthritis, generalized arthralgias, and low back pain
  - → Involves mainly large joints – especially knees
  - → Hip, wrist, hand, shoulder, and ankle are less frequently affected
- Diagnosis
  - → Psychiatric, neurologic, and hepatic disturbances are suggestive of the diagnosis
  - → Serum copper levels are elevated; ceruloplasmin levels are low
  - → 24-hour urine collection shows elevated copper excretion
  - → Genetic testing or liver biopsy is sometimes indicated
- Radiological manifestations
  - → Early OA changes – especially at knee, hip, and wrist joints
  - → Bone fragmentation and osteochondritis, especially at knee joint
  - → Chondrocalcinosis is also described
- Treatment
  - → Diet low in copper-containing foods – avoidance of mushrooms, nuts, dark chocolate, dried fruit, and shellfish
  - → D-penicillamine for copper chelation is the first described treatment
  - → Tetrathiomolybdate is employed as initial therapy to reduce free copper levels in the serum
  - → Zinc is now the mainstay of maintenance due to improved side-effect profile; it works by preventing the intestinal absorption of copper from dietary sources
- **Anatomic causes of secondary OA**
  - ○ Act by causing abnormal load distribution within the joint
  - ○ Angular misalignment is the most potent risk factor for deterioration of the joint structure because it increases the degree of focal loading
  - ○ Common anatomic abnormalities in secondary OA
    - **Slipped femoral epiphysis**
    - **Epiphyseal dysplasias**
    - **Blount's disease**
    - **Legg–Calve–Perthes disease**
    - **Congenital dislocation of the hip**
    - **Unequal leg lengths**
    - **Hypermobility syndromes**

- **Trauma and secondary OA**
  - Major joint trauma
    - Patients who have had an acute knee injury are seven times more likely to develop knee OA than are those who have not had a previous knee injury
    - Combined effect of the injury and its biomechanical consequences alter load distribution on the joint, hastening OA development
    - Anterior cruciate ligament (ACL) or meniscus tear is highly associated with knee osteoarthritis and its progression
    - Meniscus damage may play an important role in OA pathophysiology
      - Torn meniscus and extrusion seem to be strong risk factors for the development and progression of knee OA
      - Meniscectomy increases the risk of knee OA two-fold, more if combined with ACL damage or injury
      - Mixed patellofemoral and tibiofemoral OA is common in individuals who have undergone a meniscectomy

## Inflammatory/erosive hand osteoarthritis

There is controversy about inflammatory/erosive hand osteoarthritis (IE-HOA) as a separate disease entity from osteoarthritis (OA). Some characterize it as a variant of OA, a subset of OA, or an inflammatory phase of OA, while others find it an entity that is entirely distinct from OA. As a result, there is no general consensus on the definition. Typically seen in postmenopausal women, this condition poses significant diagnostic and therapeutic challenges.

### Diagnosis
- Combination of clinical and radiological features
- Some research studies use the **ACR criteria for hand OA** along with the presence of **characteristic erosions on radiography**
- EULAR description of IE-HOA
  - Characterized by an abrupt onset, marked pain and functional impairment, inflammatory symptoms and signs, including stiffness, soft tissue swelling, erythema, paresthesia, mildly elevated C-reactive protein and worse outcome than non-erosive hand OA osteoarthritis
  - Radiographically defined by subchondral erosions, cortical destruction and subsequent reparative change, which may include bony ankylosis

## Clinical features
- Abrupt onset
- Targets interphalangeal (IP) joints
  - **DIPs** more commonly involved than PIPs
  - **Second and third fingers** more commonly involved than fourth and fifth fingers, often in symmetrical fashion
- Swelling, redness, warmth, stiffness, and limited function of IP joints
- Throbbing paresthesias in finger tips
- Typically polyarticular and may persist for several years
- Accelerated progression of symptoms compared to non-erosive hand osteoarthritis
- Frequently leads to joint deformities
  - Lateral subluxations
  - Heberden's and Bouchard's nodes
  - Instability and ankylosis of DIP and PIP joints

## Radiological features
- Combination of bony proliferation and erosions seen in both DIPs and PIPs
- Joint space narrowing and erosions are seen early in the course of disease
- Later in the course – margins affected by bony proliferation lead to Heberden's and Bouchard's nodes
- **Central erosions** in subchondral bone at the articular surface are most common
  - **"Seagull-wing"** – classic appearance due to marginal sclerosis and osteophytes on the distal side of the joints while the proximal side is centrally eroded or collapsed and thinned
  - **"Saw-tooth"** – seen in PIPs

## Differential diagnosis for IE-HOA
- Nodal generalized hand OA
  - Flares mainly at onset of involvement of each joint, followed by relatively quiet disease in each individual joint
  - A stuttering pattern of polyarthropathy of DIPs and PIPs
- Psoriatic arthritis
  - Joint erosions are located more marginally, where the synovial tissue is more concentrated
  - Frequent involvement of other sites in the body (i.e. sacroiliac (SI) joints)
  - Periostitis is common in psoriatic arthritis but rare in EOA

- Rheumatoid arthritis
  - Typically involves MCPs and PIPs, sparing DIPs
  - Joint erosions are also typically more marginal

## Treatment

- To date, there is no definitive therapeutic approach to IE-HOA
- Treatments recommended for non-erosive hand osteoarthritis are frequently ineffective
  - Acetaminophen frequently inadequate, NSAIDs with limited efficacy
- Intra-articular steroid injections can provide symptomatic relief
- Hydroxychloroquine
  - Small pilot studies suggest symptomatic improvement
- Anakinra
  - Small case series with three patients suggests improvement

# Diffuse idiopathic skeletal hyperostosis (DISH)

## Introduction

- A non-inflammatory disorder, also known as **Forestier's disease** or **ankylosing hyperostosis**
- Characterized by calcification and ossification of soft tissues, mainly ligaments and where tendons and ligaments attach to bones (entheses)
  - **Hallmark of the disease – calcification of the anterolateral aspect of the thoracic spine**
- More common in people over 50 years old and men
- Etiology unknown

---

Metabolic conditions associated with DISH:
Hyperinsulinemia with or without diabetes
Obesity, especially with large waist circumference
Hyperuricemia
Dyslipidemia
Hypertension
Coronary artery disease

---

## Clinical findings

- Asymptomatic condition in many individuals
- Most common symptoms are stiffness and decreased range of spinal motion
- Mild back pain (commonly in thoracic region)

- Painful enthesopathy
- Increased susceptibility to unstable spinal fractures after trivial trauma
- Cervical spine
  - Dysphagia
  - Odynophagia and otalgia
  - Hoarseness
  - Atlantoaxial complications
  - Stridor – rare, results from large anterior osteophytes at C2–C3
  - Myelopathy – due to spinal cord compression from the posterior longitudinal ligament
- Lumbar spine
  - Radiculopathy
  - Spinal stenosis

## Radiologic findings (see also Chapter 11, Review of musculoskeletal radiology)

- Preference for axial skeleton
  - Classically involves the thoracic spine (especially the middle and lower part), but can be seen in cervical and lumbosacral spine
  - "Flowing" ossification along the anterolateral margins of vertebral bodies over four contiguous levels
    - Radiolucent line usually separates the ossified anterior longitudinal ligament from the anterior aspect of the adjacent vertebral bodies
    - Findings more prominent on right side of thoracic spine
      → Pulsation of the aorta may influence location of ossification
  - Cervical spine
    - Hyperostosis initially occurs along the anterior surface of the vertebral body
    - More common in the lower cervical spine
    - Ossification of the posterior longitudinal ligament less common, but occurs almost exclusively in the cervical spine
- Extraspinal involvement is less common, but can occur
  - Radiographic changes are often symmetric
  - Pelvis radiographs
    - Hypertrophic whiskering (bone proliferation) can involve the iliac crest, ischial tuberosity, trochanter
    - Ligament ossification
    - Periarticular osteophytes
  - Peripheral joints
    - New bone formation is prominent in the entheseal areas, particularly around the heels, knees, and elbows

- Hand – phalangeal tufting, increased cortical thickness of tubular bones of the hand, increase in the size of sesamoid bones

## Diagnosis

- Resnick and Niwayama diagnostic criteria
  - Presence of flowing calcification and ossification along the anterolateral aspects of at least four contiguous vertebral bodies
  - Preservation of the intervertebral disc spaces
  - Absence of apophyseal joint space narrowing or sacroiliac inflammatory changes

## Differential diagnosis

- Ankylosing spondylitis (AS)
  - Shared features between DISH and AS
    - Involvement of the axial skeleton and peripheral entheses
    - Bone proliferations in the latter phases of their courses
    - Both can have severe limitation of spinal mobility and postural abnormalities
  - Sacroiliac joint involvement in DISH is typically the upper, ligamentous portion
    - In AS the lower, synovial portion of the sacroiliac joint is involved
  - Peripheral enthesopathy in DISH is not as painful as in AS
  - AS begins at a younger age; it is rare for DISH to occur in patients <40 years old
  - AS is associated with inflammatory back pain symptoms
  - No SI joint erosions or bony ankylosis are noted in DISH
  - DISH has not been associated with HLA-B27
- Osteoarthritis
  - Both seen in similar age groups – both conditions may coexist
  - Distinctive features that differentiate DISH
    - Involvement of joints usually unaffected by primary OA (elbows, wrists, ankles, shoulders)
    - Increased hypertrophic changes compared with primary OA
    - Prominent enthesopathies at sites adjacent to peripheral joints
    - Calcification and ossification of entheses in sites other than joints

## Treatment

- Aimed at symptomatic relief of pain and stiffness
- Similar to OA
  - Acetaminophen
  - NSAIDs

- ○ Local applications
- ○ Physiotherapy
- ○ Weight loss
- Control of associated constitutional and metabolic disorders
- Surgery is rarely needed but can be helpful in the following settings:
  - ○ When dysphagia results from large anterior cervical osteophytes
  - ○ When progressive myelopathy results from the ossification of posterior longitudinal ligament
  - ○ In the setting of nerve root compression and thoracic outlet syndrome

## Gout

> Gout is a relatively common crystalline arthropathy that causes episodic flares of arthritis that over time may become debilitating. Deposition of excess serum uric acid crystals into an affected joint induces a subsequent local inflammatory reaction that results in characteristic pain, warmth, and swelling. This section will focus on hereditary causes of gout, as well as newer therapies in the treatment of gout.

### Causes of early-onset gout
- HGPRT (hypoxanthine-guanine phosphoribosyltransferase) deficiency
  - ○ HGPRT is a transferase enzyme that is part of the purine salvage pathway; deficiency leads to uric acid excess
  - ○ Total HGPRT deficiency => Lesch–Nyhan syndrome (X-linked recessive syndrome, mental retardation, self-mutilation, gout, nephrolithiasis)
  - ○ Partial deficiency => Kelley–Seegmiller syndrome (gout and nephrolithiasis only)
- PRPP synthetase hyperactivity
  - ○ PRPP synthetase is an enzyme necessary for de novo synthesis of purine and pyrimidine nucleotides; superactivity induces excess purine formation; subsequent catabolism of excess purines induces hyperuricemia
  - ○ Glucose-6-phosphatase (G6P) deficiency (Von Gierke's disease) is a type 1 glycogen storage disease which also induces hyperuricemia via hyperactivity of PRPP synthetase
- Polycystic kidney disease

- Familial juvenile hyperuricemic nephropathy: renal tubular disorder leads to end-stage renal disease (ESRD) by age 40 years

## Drugs causing hyperuricemia
- Thiazides
- Cyclosporine
- Ethanol
- Azathioprine: *be aware that azathioprine is metabolized by xanthine oxidase; when used in combination with allopurinol, severe leukopenia can result*
- Tacrolimus
- Nicotinic acid
- Ethambutol
- Pyrazinamide
- Warfarin
- Levodopa
- Theophylline
- Didanosine
- Loop diruetics

## Gout treatments
See Table 1.3.
- **Febuxostat** (Uloric) for the treatment of gout
  ○ As a xanthine oxidase inhibitor similar to allopurinol, febuxostat blocks the conversion of xanthine to uric acid in purine metabolism
  ○ Does not need dose adjustment in mild to moderate renal failure (CrCl >30 mL/min)
  ○ Three phase 3 randomized-controlled trials comparing febuxostat to allopurinol showed better efficacy at lowering the serum uric acid level below 6 mg/dL. Patients receiving febuxostat had an increased number of gout flares in the first 8 weeks of the medication compared to allopurinol; this equalized between groups after 8 weeks and became less frequent
  ○ Adverse events related to febuxostat in the trials included increased liver function tests (LFTs), diarrhea and dizziness
  ○ Open-label extensions of the studies found a small but increased risk of cardiovascular events in patients receiving febuxostat (2.7%) vs allopurinol (1.1%), with patients with a history of coronary atherosclerotic heart disease (CASHD) or congestive heart failure (CHF) at highest risk; therefore **febuxostat should be used in cardiac patients with caution**

**Table 1.3** Role of gout treatments for various phases of gout.

| | Treatment of acute gouty arthritis | Anti-inflammatory prophylaxis during intercritical periods | Uric acid-lowering therapy for prevention of future attacks |
|---|---|---|---|
| NSAIDS | X | | |
| Corticosteroids | X | In rare cases of gout with severe renal failure | |
| Colchicine | X | X | |
| Allopurinol | | | X |
| Febuxostat | | | X |
| Pegloticase | | | X |
| Anakinra | X | | |
| Rilonacept | X | | |

- **Pegloticase** (Krystexxa) for the treatment of gout
  - Pegloticase is a recombinant form of uricase that induces conversion of uric acid to allantoin, a metabolite that is more easily excreted by the kidney
  - Dosing is 8 mg IV q2weeks, with **no optimal duration of therapy defined**
  - Limitations
    - May precipitate gout flares due to rapid lowering of uric acid
    - Infusion reactions were common, and 5% of patients had anaphylactic reactions to the drug (vs 0 in placebo groups)
    - Must use with caution in patients with CHF, as it may precipitate CHF exacerbation
    - Study patients receiving pegloticase developed antibodies to the drug, and antibody titers were associated with decreased half-life and efficacy of drug and **increased risk of infusion reactions and anaphylaxis**
    - Contraindicated in patients with G6PD deficiency as pegloticase may precipitate hemolytic anemia

○ Clinical utility
- Utility is limited as duration of therapy has not been defined, and immunogenicity limits long-term use
- At this point, the consensus is to reserve pegloticase for patients with tophaceous gout, damaging arthropathy, and persistent gout attacks who cannot tolerate conventional treatment with allopurinol or febuxostat, or patients who do not respond to these treatments
- Anecdotal evidence shows success with using pegloticase as adjunctive therapy for 1–3 months, followed by conventional treatment with allopurinol or feboxustat, but this has not been studied
- The ACR recommends checking a serum uric acid level prior to each pegloticase infusion; if the uric acid level during treatment rises to above 6 mg/dL, consider discontinuing pegloticase as this may predict risk of infusion reactions and anaphylaxis
- Antibodies to pegloticase may be checked as well to follow immunogenicity, but this testing is expensive and not widely available

- **Rasburicase** for the treatment of gout
  ○ Although it is useful in preventing renal failure in hyperuricemia due to tumor lysis syndrome, its use in treatment in non-oncologic indications is limited
  ○ Rasburicase has a short half-life (less than 24 hours) and may induce severe hypersensitivity reactions in as many as 5% of patients
  ○ Immunogenicity is also a concern that limits long-term efficacy
  ○ One study from 2002 randomized gout patients that could not receive allopurinol treatment to rasburicase once monthly for 6 months or once daily for 5 days
    - Methylprednisolone was infused as a pretreatment for every infusion of rasburicase
    - Patients receiving monthly rasburicase had lower serum uric acid levels and 2/5 patients had reduction in tophi size
    - Patients receiving daily rasburicase did not have improvements in either serum uric acid concentrations or tophi
    - Patients still had increased gout attacks during the study period; adverse events including hypersensitivity reactions were common
  ○ Given hypersensitivity, immunogenicity, and short half-life, rasburicase remains a drug with primarily oncologic indications

- **Anakinra** for the treatment of gout
  ○ Anakinra is an IL-1 inhibitor approved for the treatment of rheumatoid arthritis
  ○ It is a recombinant human IL-1 receptor antagonist that inhibits both membrane-bound and circulating IL-1 isoforms

○ The basis for IL-1 inhibition in the treatment of acute gout stems from animal data showing uric acid as a key trigger of inflammasome activity and production of IL-1B, making acute gout a disease potentially mediated by IL-1B

○ Anakinra and gout open-label pilot study:
- Patients with acute gout who failed conventional treatment received daily anakinra for 3 days
- Nine of ten patients had complete resolution of acute gout by day 3

○ The bottom line: further studies need to be done to confirm the results of the initial study; additionally, although rapid response to anakinra may warrant its use in some cases, at this point its cost limits regular use in all patients

- **Rilonacept** for the treatment of gout
   ○ Building on data for inflammasome and IL-1B activity in gout, rilonacept as an alternate IL-1 inhibitor to anakinra is gaining attention
   ○ Rilonacept was originally produced and recently approved for treatment of CAPS (cryopyrin-associated periodic syndromes); it is a recombinant protein that binds IL-1A and IL-1B preventing their binding and activation to the IL-1 receptor complex
   ○ A pilot study of 10 patients with chronic gout receiving weekly rilonacept for 6 weeks showed improvement in pain scores and inflammatory markers at 2, 4, and 6 weeks of follow up
   ○ Further study is warranted to determine if IL-1 inhibition will be a valid and effective additional gout treatment strategy

## Further reading

Bacconnier, L. et al. (2009) Erosive osteoarthritis of the hand: clinical experience with subcutaneous injection of anakinra. *Annals of the Rheumatic Diseases* 68: 1078–1079.

Bryant, LR. et al. (1995) Hydroxychloroquine in the treatment of erosive osteoarthritis. *Journal of Rheumatology* 22: 1527–1531.

Campbell, J., Bellamy, N., Gee, T. (2007) Differences between systematic reviews/meta-analyses of hyaluronic acid/hyaluronan/hylan in osteoarthritis of the knee. *Osteoarthritis and Cartilage* 15: 1424–1436.

Hochberg, M. et al. (2012) American College of Rheumatology 2012 Recommendations for the use of nonpharmacologic and pharmacologic therapies in osteoarthritis of the hand, hip and knee. *Arthritis Care & Research* 64(4) 465–474.

Jordan, K.M. et al. (2003) EULAR Recommendations 2003: An evidence based approach to the management of knee osteoarthritis: report of a task force of the EULAR Standing Committee for International Clinical Studies Including Therapeutic Trials (ESCISIT). *Annals of Rheumatic Disease* 62: 1145–1155.

Oliveri, I. et al. (2009) Diffuse idiopathic skeletal hyperostosis: differentiation from ankylosing spondylitis. *Current Rheumatology Reports* 11: 321–328.

Resnick, D. et al. (1976) Radiographic and pathologic features of spinal involvement in diffuse idiopathic skeletal hyperostosis (DISH). *Radiology* 119: 559–568.

Rutjes, A.W., Juni, P., de Costa, B.R., et al. (2012) Viscosupplementation for osteoarthritis of the knee: a systematic review and meta-analysis. *Annals of Internal Medicine* 157(3): 180–191.

Sarzi-Puttini, P. et al. (2004) New developments in our understanding of DISH (diffuse idiopathic skeletal hyperostosis). *Current Opinion In Rheumatology* 16: 287–292.

Zhang, W. et al. (2007) EULAR evidence based recommendations for the management of hand osteoarthritis: report of a task force of the EULAR Standing Committee for International Clinical Studies Including Therapeutics (ESCISIT). *Annals of Rheumatic Disease* 66: 377–388.

Zhang, W. et al. (2005) EULAR evidence based recommendations for the management of hip osteoarthritis: report of a task force of the EULAR Standing Committee for International Clinical Studies Including Therapeutics (ESCISIT). *Annals of Rheumatic Disease* 64: 669–681.

Zhang, W. et al. (2008) OARSI Recommendations for the Management of Hip and Knee Osteoarthritis, Part II: OARSI evidence-based, expert consensus guidelines. *Osteoarthritis and Cartilage* 16: 137–162.

# CHAPTER 2

# Selected topics in rheumatoid arthritis

**Athan Tiliakos, Karen Law, Aliza Lipson**

Emory University School of Medicine, Atlanta, GA, USA

## Introduction

The field of rheumatoid arthritis (RA) continues to expand, especially with the establishment of updated classification criteria, application of more specific serologies in diagnosis, understanding of broader systemic issues related to the disease, and new medications able to offer additional treatment options for patients who fail standard therapy. These major developments are reviewed in this chapter.

## 2010 ACR/EULAR RA classification criteria

- In an effort to identify early stages of disease, the American College of Rheumatology (ACR) and the European League Against Rheumatism (EULAR) collaborated and developed new classification criteria for RA
- These new 2010 criteria replace the previously developed 1987 American Rheumatism Association's Criteria
- The 2010 ACR/EULAR criteria include **joint involvement** (both size and number of joints), the presence and titers of **rheumatoid factor** (RF) or anti-citrullinated antibodies (ACPAs), the presence of **elevated acute phase reactants**, and the **duration of symptoms**. Each of these criteria is given a score, with a total value of greater than or equal to 6/10 being required for the diagnosis of "definite RA"

---

*Rheumatology Board Review*, First Edition. Edited by Karen Law and Aliza Lipson.
© 2014 John Wiley & Sons, Inc. Published 2014 by John Wiley & Sons, Inc.

○ The criteria can be applied if the patient has **at least one joint with synovitis**, and the synovitis cannot be better explained by another disease

○ Small joint involvement as well as >10 joints involved are scored higher, increasing the likelihood of RA, *however*, DIPs, first CMC, and first MTP joints are excluded from assessment

---

**Keep in mind**

The DIPs are typically spared in RA, and the first CMC and MTP joints are more commonly affected by osteoarthritis.

---

○ Joint "involvement" is defined as either **tenderness** or **swelling**

○ Duration of symptoms >6 weeks is scored higher, increasing the likelihood of RA

○ Patients with a high suspicion for RA who do not score 6 or greater on initial assessment may also fulfill the criteria prospectively, highlighting the cumulative nature of joint manifestations in RA

• In keeping with the theme of identifying RA in the early stages, the 2010 Classification criteria **do not include** the 1987 criteria of morning stiffness, rheumatoid nodules, and radiographic changes

• By focusing on identifying RA in early stages, experts caution that the criteria are for **classification**, not diagnosis, may have low specificity in clinical practice, and may incorrectly label patients as having RA instead of another inflammatory arthritis

## Anti-citrullinated antibodies

### What are they?

• In order to fully understand the significance of anti-citrullinated antibodies (ACPAs), it is important to understand the process of citrullination

• Citrullination is facilitated by enzymes called peptidyl arginine deiminases (PADs), in an environment of high calcium concentrations; PADs are able to post-translationally modify arginines into citrullines

• During apoptosis, the process of citrullination is thought to assist in the breakdown of intracellular proteins

○ Normally, the breakdown products are removed by cells involved in the clearance of apoptotic debris

○ In situations where apoptotic cell clearance is impaired, extracellular proteins may be exposed to PADs, which can lead to further citrullination and potential antibody formation
- ACPA formation requires more than the mere presence of citrullinated proteins
   ○ Genetic factors (i.e. shared epitope) and environmental factors (smoking) can lead to the increased risk of developing ACPA

## What is the role of ACPA in the diagnosis of RA?
- ACPA formation may precede clinical disease by several years
- Studies have shown that the sensitivity of ACPA and rheumatoid factor (RF) are comparable, but the specificity of ACPAs is favorable when compared to RF in diagnosing RA
- Importantly, ACPA is not typically present in hepatitis C, while RF is frequently elevated in hepatitis C

---

**Elevated RF may be seen in:**
Hepatitis B or C
Human immunodeficiency virus (HIV) infection
Syphilis
Endocarditis
Tuberculosis (TB)
Leprosy
Schistosomiasis

---

- The presence of ACPA has been shown to signal a worse disease prognosis as evidenced by more severe joint destruction, and extra-articular manifestations of RA

## Rheumatoid arthritis and cardiovascular disease

- Patients with RA are at an increased risk for developing cardiovascular (CV) disease
- It has been reported that the risk of cardiovascular disease in RA patients appears to be similar to those without RA who are 10 years older
- This increased risk appears to be **independent** of the traditional risk factors for CV disease
- Several studies have shown that when the traditional CV risk factors have been adjusted for, **increased systemic inflammation** and **disease activity/severity** correlate with increased risk of cardiovascular events

- It is important to look at some of the traditional risk factors of CV disease and see how they relate to patients with RA
  - Hypertension
    - Studies have shown that hypertension is common in RA, but the prevalence does not seem to be greater when compared to control groups without RA
    - Certain medications (e.g. NSAIDs), obesity, and inactivity of patients secondary to joint damage or active disease are some of the factors that may provide challenges to appropriately treating hypertension in patients with RA
  - Dyslipidemia
    - Multiple studies have shown that when compared to the general population, patients with RA may have lower levels of total cholesterol, low-density lipoprotein (LDL), and high-density lipoprotein (HDL).
    - In fact, Myasoedova et al. demonstrated that total cholesterol and LDH levels significantly decreased in the 5 years prior to the diagnosis of RA
  - Diabetes mellitus (DM) and metabolic syndrome
    - In a 2011 meta-analysis, Boyer et al. found that there was an increased prevalence of DM in patients with RA when compared to controls
    - Multiple studies have shown an increased prevalence of the metabolic syndrome in patients with RA

## Treatment advances in rheumatoid arthritis

New medications for the treatment of RA have undergone rapid expansion in the last decade, primarily in the group of drugs known as biologics, or biologic response modifiers. These medications all share a common origin as genetically engineered proteins derived from human genes. Each targets a specific component of the immune system to reduce the inflammation associated with RA. Biologics have revolutionized the treatment of RA, particularly for patients with moderate to severe RA who do not respond adequately to traditional disease-modifying antirheumatic drugs (DMARDs). The first biologic medications developed were the tumor necrosis factor (TNF) inhibitors, including etanercept, adalimumab, and infliximab. Newer medications with novel mechanisms of action have since been introduced, and will be reviewed here.

## Anakinra – approved 2001
- Anakinra is an IL-1 receptor antagonist that **blocks the proinflammatory activity of IL-1** by competing for its binding sites
- By blocking the effects of IL-1, anakinra reduces B and T cell activation, cytokine production, synovial proliferation, and cartilage and bone destruction typically mediated by IL-1
- Anakinra is administered subcutaneously once daily, and has been shown to have moderate efficacy in RA when compered to placebo; it has also been shown to inhibit radiographic progression
- Experts do point out that while studies show that patients do improve on anakinra, those improvements are modest compared to other biologics: ACR20 response rates in the five original randomized–control trials ranged from 38–42%
- Based on these studies, anakinra is approved for use in RA patients who have had inadequate response to conventional disease-modifying treatment
- Safety issues
  - Importantly, there was no increase in infection risk associated with anakinra
  - The most common adverse events were mild injection site reactions, including erythema, rash, and itching
  - Lack of widespread use has been largely due to the prevalence of injection site reactions and the requirement for daily injections

## Abatacept – approved 2006
- Abatacept is a fusion protein comprised of the Fc portion of human IgG and the extracellular domain of CTLA-4
- Abatacept binds the B7 protein on antigen-presenting cells with high affinity, and thereby **blocks the CD28:B7 costimulatory binding signal** required for full T cell activation
- Abatacept is administered intravenously every 4 weeks, and has been shown to be superior to methotrexate alone after 12 months of treatment; studies in patients with inadequate response to anti-TNFs showed similar improvement after treatment with abatacept
- Based on these studies, it is approved for use in RA patients who have had inadequate response to methotrexate or anti-TNFs
- Safety issues
  - Increased risk of serious infections, though no opportunistic infections have been reported in studies to date; routine screening for latent TB infection prior to treatment start is recommended

○ Increased exacerbations and infections in patients with chronic obstructive pulmonary disease (COPD)
• Recently, a self-administered weekly subcutaneous formulation of abatacept has been approved, with similar efficacy and toxicity profile to the intravenous formulation

## Rituximab – approved 2006

• Rituximab is a monoclonal antibody directed against CD20 proteins expressed on the surface of B cells
• Rituximab **depletes B cells that express CD20** from the peripheral blood, thereby reducing autoantibody and immune complex production as well as T cell stimulation and cytokine production involved in inflammation from RA
• Rituximab is administered intravenously on days 1 and 15, with retreatment after 6 months or longer
  ○ Specific recommendations on the interval of retreatment have not yet been established
• Studies show rituximab and rituximab plus methotrexate to be superior to methotrexate alone in patients with inadequate response to methotrexate; similar results were reported in patients with inadequate response to anti-TNFs
• Clinical responses were of longer duration when rituximab is used in combination with methotrexate
• Based on these studies, rituximab is approved for use in patients with inadequate response to anti-TNFs
• At this point, there is no established protocol for checking peripheral B cell counts (CD19 cells) or immunoglobulin levels before or after rituximab treatment, to determine response to therapy or time to retreatment
  ○ Early data suggest that complete B cell depletion correlates with increased response to the drug, so monitoring may have utility in this regard
• Safety issues
  ○ Slight increased risk of serious infections, though no opportunistic infections have been reported in studies to date; routine screening for latent TB infection prior to treatment start is not required
  ○ Infusion reactions are common and typically improve with subsequent infusions; acetaminophen, diphenhydramine, and pretreatment corticosteroids can be helpful
  ○ Fatal infusion reactions have been reported in four patients receiving rituximab for RA

○ Case reports in patients with lymphoma, lupus, or RA treated with rituximab suggest a small but increased risk of progressive multifocal leukoencephalopathy (PML), however the long-term overall risk of PML in patients receiving rituximab for RA or other rheumatic diseases is unknown

## Tocilizumab – approved 2010

• Tocilizumab is a monoclonal antibody directed against the IL-6 receptor
• Tocilizumab **blocks the proinflammatory functions of IL-6**, including the stimulation of T and B cells and macrophages to promote the transition from acute to chronic inflammation
• Tocilizumab is administered intravenously every 4 weeks, and has been shown to be superior to methotrexate in studies of methotrexate-naïve patients; it has also been shown to be superior in inadequate responders to methotrexate or anti-TNFs
• Based on these studies, it is approved for use either in combination with methotrexate, or as monotherapy, for patients who have had inadequate response to anti-TNFs
• Safety issues
  ○ Like other biologics, tocilizumab carries an **increased risk of serious bacterial, invasive fungal, mycobacterial, and opportunistic infections**; all patients should be screened for latent TB prior to starting the medication
  ○ **Neutropenia, thrombocytopenia**, and **liver enzyme elevation** have been reported; dose reduction is recommended in these situations
  ○ **Increased incidence of gastrointestinal (GI) perforations** were noted in patients receiving tocilizumab, typically colonic perforations in the setting of known diverticulitis, though upper GI perforation did occur in two patients
  ○ **Lipid profile abnormalities** were noted including elevated total cholesterol, LDL, HDL, and triglycerides; routine lipid monitoring is recommended while on tocilizumab though guidelines for initiation of lipid-lowering medications in this setting have not been established
  ○ Tocilizumab has not been studied and is not recommended for patients with hepatitis B or hepatitis C infection, patients with creatinine clearance <50 mL/min, or patients with transaminases >1.5× upper limit of normal

# Appropriate immunizations and screening in RA patients

## Tuberculosis screening

- Screen to identify LTBI (latent TB infection) in **all RA patients** being considered for use of a biologic agent, regardless of the presence or absence of risk factors
- Risk factors for TB (CDC guidelines)
  - Close contacts of persons known or suspected to have active TB
  - Foreign-born persons from areas that have high incidence of active TB (Africa, Asia, eastern Europe, Latin America, Russia)
  - Persons who visit areas with high prevalence of active TB, especially if for frequent or prolonged visits
  - Residents and employees of congregate settings whose clients are at an increased risk for active TB (correctional facilities, long-term care facilities, homeless shelters)
  - Healthcare workers who serve clients who are at an increased risk for active TB
  - Populations defined locally as having increased incidence of LTBI or active TB (possibly including medically underserved, low-income populations or persons who abuse drugs/alcohol)
  - Infants, children, and adolescents exposed to adults who are at an increased risk of LTBI or active TB
- Options for screening for LTBI
  - Tuberculin skin test (TST)
  - Interferon-gamma-release assays (IGRAs) – preferred if there is a history of BCG vaccination
    - If TST or IGRA is positive or if clinically indicated for another reason, obtain chest x-ray
    - If chest x-ray is positive, obtain sputum for AFB (acid-fast bacilli) to rule out active TB (may require specialist referral)
    - For LTBI or active TB, refer to an infectious diseases specialist or the Health Department for treatment
- Timing of biologics when TB is present
  - LTBI: complete treatment for LTBI **for 1 month prior** to staring biologic therapy
  - Active TB: complete treatment for active TB prior to starting biologic therapy

A positive TST or IGRA may remain positive, even after treatment. Patients must be monitored clinically and evaluated for reinfection with chest x-ray and sputum studies, based on clinical suspicion.

## Key points in using vaccines in RA patients

- Vaccines should be administered based on individual patient age and risk (Table 2.1)
- Pneumococcal vaccination:
  - The CDC recommends receipt of the vaccine for RA patients, and a one-time pneumococcal revaccination after 5 years
  - Additionally, patients who receive the pneumococcal vaccine (PCV23) before age 65 years should receive revaccination after age 65 once, at least 5 years after initial vaccination
  - New recommendations promote the use of the PCV13 form of the pneumococcal vaccine, traditionally used in children <5 years of age, for improved immune response
  - These guidelines recommend the use of PCV13 as the initial pneumococcal vaccine for immunocompromised patients, followed by PCV23 8 weeks later, with resumption of the traditional revaccination schedule thereafter, however these recommendations have yet to be fully incorporated into routine medical practice
- Hepatitis B vaccine
  - Hepatitis B vaccine should be given if risk factors are present, including intravenous drug use, multiple sex partners in the previous 6 months, or if the patient is a healthcare worker
- Herpes zoster (shingles) vaccine
  - Patients with RA and other autoimmune diseases have 1.5–2-fold increased risk of developing shingles

**Table 2.1** Summary of suggested vaccine schedule for RA patients.

| | Killed vaccines <br> • Pneumococcal pneumonia <br> • Influenza (intramuscular) <br> • Hepatitis B | Recombinant vaccine <br> • Human papillomavirus | Live attenuated vaccine <br> • Herpes zoster |
|---|---|---|---|
| Before starting treatment with **DMARDs** | + | + | + |
| Before starting biologics | + | + | + |
| While on **current** treatment with **DMARDs** | + | + | + |
| While on **current** treatment with **biologics** | + | + | X |

**Table 2.2** Summary of drug toxicity monitoring in RA patients.

| | Baseline | Complete blood count, liver enzymes, creatinine | | |
| --- | --- | --- | --- | --- |
| | | <3 months | 3–6 months | >6 months |
| Hydroxychloroquine | + | Baseline | None | None |
| Leflunomide | + | 2–4 weeks | 8–12 weeks | 12 weeks |
| Methotrexate | + | 2–4 weeks | 8–12 weeks | 12 weeks |
| Minocycline | + | Baseline | None | None |
| Sulfasalazine | + | 2–4 weeks | 8–12 weeks | 12 weeks |

Hepatitis B and C screening is recommended prior to starting leflunomide and methotrexate (if risk factors exist)
Ophthalmologic exam is recommended within the first year of treatment with hydroxychloroquine, and every 1–2 years thereafter while on treatment

    ○ As a live vaccine, patients should receive it prior to starting biologics for RA; they can receive it if on non-biologic DMARD therapy
    ○ It is not recommended for those already taking biologic therapy (although temporarily holding biologic therapy to give the vaccine may be considered)
    ○ Effectiveness studies suggest the vaccine is as effective in patients with RA
    ○ Because the duration of long-term immunity from an episode of shingles is not known, most infectious diseases specialists recommend vaccination regardless of if the patient has recently manifested with shingles

## Drug toxicity monitoring
See Table 2.2.

## Further reading

Aletaha, D., Neogi, T., Silman, A.J., et al. (2010) Rheumatoid Arthritis Classification Criteria: An American College of Rheumatology/European League Against Rheumatism collaborative initiative. *Arthritis and Rheumatism* 62: 2569–2581.

American College of Rheumatology (2012) Update of the 2008 American College of Rheumatology Recommendations for the use of disease-modifying antirheumatic drugs and biologic agents in the treatment of rheumatoid arthritis. *Arthritis Care and Research* 64(5): 625–639.

American College of Rheumatology (2008) Recommendations for the use of nonbiologic and biologic disease-modifying antirheumatic drugs in rheumatoid arthritis. *Arthritis Care and Research* (59)6: 762–784

Boyer, J.-F., Gourraud, P.A. Cantagrel, A., et al. (2011) Traditional cardiovascular risk factors in rheumatoid arthritis: a meta-analysis. *Joint Bone Spine* 78: 179–183.

Cohen, S.B., Greenwald, M., Dougadas, M.R., et al. (2005) Efficacy and safety of rituximab in active RA patients who experience an inadequate response to one or more anti-TNF therapies (REFLEX Study). *Arthritis and Rheumatism* 52(suppl): S677.

Cohen, S., Hurd, E., Cush, J., et al. (2002) Treatment of rheumatoid arthritis with anakinra, a recombinant human interleukin-1 receptor antagonist, in combination with methotrexate: results of a twenty-four-week, multicenter, randomized, double-blind, placebo-controlled trial. *Arthritis and Rheumatism* 46(3): 614–624.

Cohen, S., Moreland, L., Cush, J., et al. (2004) A multicentre, double blind, randomised, placebo controlled trial of anakinra (Kineret), a recombinant interleukin 1 receptor antagonist, in patients with rheumatoid arthritis treated with background methotrexate. *Annals of the Rheumatic Diseases* 63(9): 1062–1068.

Edwards, J.C., Szczepanski, L., Szechinski, J., et al. (2004) Efficacy of B-cell targeted therapy with rituximab in patients with rheumatoid arthritis. *New England Journal of Medicine* 350: 2572–2781.

Emery, P., Fleischmann, R., Filipowicz-Sosnowska, A., et al. (2006) The efficacy and safety of rituximab in patients with active rheumatoid arthritis despite methotrexate treatment: results of a phase iib randomized, double-blind, placebo-controlled, dose-ranging trial. *Arthritis and Rheumatism* 54: 1390–1400.

Gabriel, S. and Crowson, C. (2012) Risk factors for cardiovascular disease in rheumatoid arthritis. *Current Opinion in Rheumatology* 24: 171–176.

Genovese, M.C., Becker, J.-C., Schiff, M., et al. (2005) Abatacept for rheumatoid arthritis refractory to tumor necrosis factor in inhibition. *New England Journal of Medicine* 353: 1114–1123.

Genovese, M.C., McKay, J.D., Nasonov, E.L., et al. (2008) Interleukin-6 receptor inhibition with tocilizumab reduces disease activity in rheumatoid arthritis with inadequate response to disease-modifying antirheumatic drugs: the tocilizumab in combination with traditional disease-modifying antirheumatic drug therapy study. *Arthritis and Rheumatism* 58(10): 2968–2980.

Gonzalez, A., Maradit Kremers, H., Crowson, C.S., et al. (2008) Do cardiovascular risk factors confer the same risk for cardiovascular outcomes in rheumatoid arthritis patients as in non-rheumatoid arthritis patients? *Annals of the Rheumatic Diseases* 67: 64–69.

Maini, R.N., Taylor, P.C., Szechinski, J., et al. (2006) Double-blind randomized controlled clinical trial of the interleukin-6 receptor antagonist, tocilizumab, in European patients with rheumatoid arthritis who had an incomplete response to methotrexate. *Arthritis and Rheumatism* 54(9): 2817–2829.

Myasoedova, E., Crowson, C.S., Kremers, H.M., et al. (2010) Total cholesterol and LDL levels decrease before rheumatoid arthritis. *Annals of the Rheumatic Diseases* 69: 1310–1314.

Rantapaa-Dahlqvist, S., de Jong, B.A.W., Berglin, E., et al. (2003) Antibodies against cyclic citrullinated peptide and IgA rheumatoid factor predict the development of rheumatoid arthritis. *Arthritis and Rheumatism* 48: 2741–2749.

Smolen, J.S., Beaulieu, A., Rubbert-Roth, A., et al. (2008) Effect of interleukin-6 receptor inhibition with tocilizumab in patients with rheumatoid arthritis (OPTION study): a double-blind, placebo-controlled, randomised trial. *Lancet* 371(9617): 987–997.

Snow, M. and Mikuls, T. (2005) Rheumatoid arthritis and cardiovascular disease: the role of systemic inflammation and evolving strategies of prevention. *Current Opinion in Rheumatology* 17: 234–241.

Van Gaalen, F.A., Linn-Rasker, S.P., van Venrooij, W.J., et al. (2004) Autoantibodies to cyclic citrullinated peptides predict progression to rheumatoid arthritis in patients with undifferentiated arthritis: a prospective cohort study. *Arthritis and Rheumatism* 50: 709–715.

Van der Linden, M.P.M., Knevel, R., Huizinga, T.W., et al. (2011) Classification of rheumatoid arthritis. Comparison of the 1987 American College of Rheumatology Criteria and the 2010 American College of rheumatology/European League Against Rheumatism Criteria. *Arthritis and Rheumatism* 63: 37–42.

CHAPTER 3

# Selected topics in systemic lupus erythematosus: B cells in lupus and lupus nephritis

**Iñaki Sanz, S. Sam Lim**

Emory University School of Medicine, Atlanta, GA, USA

## Introduction

B cells contribute to the pathogenesis of systemic lupus erythematosus (SLE) through multiple actions, including primary autoantibody production as well as antigen presentation, T cell induction, and the secretion of proinflammatory cytokines. Therefore, the development of biologic therapies designed to target B cells in SLE has remained of great interest to researchers. This chapter will review the rationale for B cells as therapeutic targets in SLE, as well as several key trials investigating the efficacy of these biologic agents in treating SLE. Additionally, the classification, treatment, and monitoring of lupus nephritis, one of the most problematic manifestations of SLE, will be reviewed.

## B cell roles in SLE

• Autoantibody production results in the formation of immune complexes that accumulate in tissues, inducing a **type III hypersensitivity reaction** that manifests clinically as nephritis, arthritis, and other disease manifestations

*Rheumatology Board Review*, First Edition. Edited by Karen Law and Aliza Lipson.
© 2014 John Wiley & Sons, Inc. Published 2014 by John Wiley & Sons, Inc.

○ Autoantibody-producing cells fall into two categories: **short-lived** and **long-lived populations** which have differing CD20 expression and antibody production profiles

○ This separation bears important implications for our understanding of SLE pathogenesis

○ Rational design of therapeutic strategies must take into account the markers differentially expressed by short-lived and long-lived plasma cells, as well as the roles of different classes of autoantibodies

- Immune complexes, perhaps more powerfully those formed by anti-ribonucleoprotein antibodies, also induce disease due to their ability to co-engage stimulatory **Fcγ receptors** and **Toll-like receptors** (TLRs) in dendritic cells, thereby promoting the production of type I interferon and amplification of inflammation

- **Additional antibody-independent functions** are increasingly recognized as contributing significantly to disease pathogenesis, including:

○ Promotion of CD4+ and CD8+ effector T cell populations including $T_H17$ induction

○ Inhibition of $T_{REG}$ cell populations

○ Recruitment of dendritic cells

○ Production of proinflammatory cytokines including TNF and IL-6

- Of note, **B cells can also suppress autoimmunity** through a variety of functions that often represent the mirror image of their pathogenic functions; whether this balancing act represents a competition between different B cell subsets with a committed phenotype to a given function or instead is achieved by environmental modulation of multi-functional cells remains to be elucidated

- **B cells suppress autoimmunity** through the following functions:

○ Induction of T cell anergy

○ Suppression of helper T cells

○ Expansion of $T_{REG}$ cell populations

○ Inhibition of dendritic cells

○ Production of anti-inflammatory cytokines, predominantly IL-10

  ▪ In humans, both transitional B cells and B10 cells (regulatory B cells that produce IL-10) have been shown to be able to downregulate $T_H$ cell activation and reduce the production of proinflammatory cytokines by monocytes through the production of IL-10

  ▪ Of significant interest, transitional regulatory B cells, while numerically increased, have been postulated to be functionally deficient in SLE

  ▪ Similarly, B10 cells and their precursors can also be increased in active SLE, suggesting either a functional deficiency or increased resistance of their target cells

# Therapies targeting B cells

Strategic, selective B cell targeting through therapies that either promote B cell suppression of autoimmunity or inhibit B cell autoantibody production and antibody-independent autoimmunity have a pathologic basis for utility in the treatment of SLE.

## Specific approaches
- **Direct B cell depletion** through depleting antibodies (rituximab)
- **Interference with B cell survival** and **enforcement of B cell tolerance** during early B cell differentiation (belimumab)
- **Inhibition of cytokines** known to play an important role in the differentiation and/or survival of memory B cells and plasma cells (IL-21, type 1 interferon, and IL-6)
- **Interruption of B cell receptor signaling** or B cell costimulatory receptors including TLRs
- **Engagement of B cell inhibitory receptors**
  - If associated with linked recognition of autoantigens, this strategy could theoretically lead to specific inhibition of pathogenic B cells
- **Expansion of regulatory B cells**, accomplished either in vivo or in vitro with subsequent reinfusion of expanded regulatory B cells

## Existing therapies for SLE

### Rituximab
- Infusion of rituximab, an anti-CD20 antibody, mediates cell death in all B cells that express CD20 by a combination of mechanisms that include ADCC (antibody-dependent cell-mediated cytotoxicity), complement-mediated cytotoxicity, and direct induction of apoptosis
- The **EXPLORER** and **LUNAR** trials are two multicenter, randomized trials of rituximab in moderate to severe active SLE
  - EXPLORER examined moderate to severe, active, non-renal SLE patients receiving either rituximab or placebo in addition to steroids and stable background immunosuppressive therapy
  - LUNAR examined class II/IV, active lupus nephritis receiving rituximab or placebo in addition to mycophenolate mofetil
  - Neither trial was able to show that the addition of rituximab in these patients was superior to placebo when added to standard of care
- Given the reported benefit of rituximab in clinical practice in off-label use, these results have been disappointing to researchers; many feel that the diversity of disease among patients and difficulty designing a study

to assess a multisystem, heterogeneous disease process are to blame for the lack of evidence of benefit
- There are several additional considerations tied specifically to rituximab that are currently under study
  - Pre-specified subset analyses in the EXPLORER trial have shown benefit in African-American and Hispanic patients
  - Similar analysis of the LUNAR trial also showed clinical benefit in African-American nephritis patients, although the small numbers of such patients in the study precluded more definitive conclusions
  - Also of significant importance, the primary endpoint of LUNAR failed to incorporate patients with partial renal remission, a clinical outcome of substantial relevance that is likely to portend long-term outcomes
  - Neither trial analyzed if complete B cell depletion occurred in each patient receiving rituximab; lower depletion levels have been shown to correlate with increased response to the drug
    - Thus, these studies cannot differentiate between lack of benefit from complete B cell depletion and failure to achieve this immunological outcome

## Belimumab
- Belimumab is a monoclonal antibody that binds to and inhibits BLys, a soluble B lymphocyte stimulator (also known as BAFF), that is necessary for B cell survival
  - In addition, excess BAFF, a common SLE abnormality, promotes the survival and maturation of immature and naïve B cells, thereby contributing to the accumulation of these cells in the mature peripheral compartment
- **BLISS-52** and **BLISS-76** are two recent, large-scale, phase III clinical trials of belimumab for the treatment of SLE whose success led to the FDA approval of this drug for the treatment of SLE
  - Both used the SLE Responder Index (SRI) as the measure of the primary efficacy endpoint; this index was designed specifically for use in these trials
  - Results from both trials showed that belimumab modestly reduced disease activity and increased time to flare compared to placebo as well as reduced the need for corticosteroid treatment
    - BLISS-52: SRI response rate of 58% for belimumab, 44% for placebo at 52 weeks (10 mg/kg; $p = 0.0006$)
    - BLISS-76: SRI response rate of 43% for belimumab, 34% for placebo at 52 weeks (10 mg/kg; $p = 0.017$)

↪ Of note, BLISS-76 did not show superiority for lower doses of belimumab (1 mg/kg; p = 0.089) in contrast to BLISS-52 (p = 0.0129)

↪ BLISS-76 was performed in western Europe and North America, while BLISS-52 was carried out in eastern Europe and Asia

○ Belimumab was not associated with increased rates of serious infection

○ Belimumab has not yet been studied in patients with severe, active lupus nephritis or CNS lupus

○ Few African-Americans were included in BLISS-76

---

Belimumab is the first new medication to be FDA approved for the treatment of SLE in over 50 years, and has generated much interest regarding proof-of-principle in targeting B cells in the treatment of SLE.

• Additional important questions remain to be investigated

○ The optimal timing of belimumab treatment in an individual patient's disease course

○ If certain individual patient characteristics may be more responsive to belimumab based on disease manifestations, ethnicity, or immunologic markers

• Conversely, the benefit of this modality in patients with renal disease and African-Americans remains to be established

The current data, observational experience, and the immunological basis for this approach suggest that BAFF blockade might play an important synergistic role when added to B cell depletion (known to increase available BAFF levels) for remission induction as well as maintenance therapy.

---

## Additional therapies targeting B cells in SLE under investigation

• **Atacicept**, a recombinant TACI-FC receptor fusion protein capable of binding to both BLyS as well as APRIL, a cytokine that powerfully mediates memory B cell and plasma cell survival, impacts the survival of a broader swath of B cells and plasma cells and has a more powerful effect on antibody titers

○ The promise of this agent has been compromised by the occurrence of serious infectious complications that led to the interruption of clinical trials both in rheumatoid arthritis and SLE (the latter when combined with mycophenolate mofetil)

- **Epratuzumab** is an anti-CD22 antibody that inhibits B cell activation and maturation and induces a more modest degree of B cell depletion
    - ○ Early, small studies show a steroid-sparing effect at 24 weeks
- **Bortezomib** is a proteosome inhibitor commonly used to treat multiple myeloma
    - ○ By selectively inhibiting the 26s proteasome, resulting in apoptosis, bortezomib has shown promise in triggering plasma cell apoptosis and modifying the proinflammatory response
    - ○ Dramatic improvement of lupus nephritis has been demonstrated with this agent in mouse models
    - ○ The unique mechanism of action of this class of agents, the importance of autoantibody-producing plasma cells (not directly affected by rituximab or belimumab) and the availability of new-generation proteasome inhibitors (such as carfilzomib) with significantly reduced incidence of painful peripheral neuropathy, all illustrate the promise of this approach for the treatment of SLE

## Lupus nephritis

Lupus nephritis (LN) can run the clinical gamut from mild proteinuria to severe glomerulonephritis with nephrotic range proteinuria leading to end-stage renal disease. Involvement can include the glomerulus, tubulointerstitium, and/or vasculature. It is estimated that 35% of adults with systemic lupus erythematosus have clinical evidence of some form of lupus nephritis, with upwards of 60% developing nephritis some time during the first 10 years of disease.

### Classification criteria
- Beginning with the original 1974 WHO Classification, classification of lupus nephritis has been based entirely on glomerular involvement
- The most recent classification system was published in 2004 and is called the International Society of Nephrology/Renal Pathology Society (ISN/RPS) 2003 Classification of Lupus Nephritis (Table 3.1)
- Definitions adopted were based on light microscopy and immunofluorescence findings – electron microscopy was excluded due to lack of worldwide access
    - ○ Subcategories of membranous lupus nephritis class V denoting coexistent membranous and proliferative disease were eliminated and replaced with lupus nephritis class IV and V, reducing the chance of

**Table 3.1** ISN/RPS (2003) Classification of Lupus Nephritis.

| Class | Description |
|---|---|
| Class I | Minimal mesangial lupus nephritis |
| Class II | Mesangial proliferative lupus nephritis |
| Class III | Focal lupus nephritis[a] (<50% of glomeruli)<br>III (A): active lesions<br>III (A/C): active and chronic lesions<br>III (C): chronic lesions |
| Class IV | Diffuse lupus nephritis[b] (≥50% of glomeruli)<br>Diffuse segmental (IV-S) or global (IV-G) lupus nephritis<br>IV (A): active lesions<br>IV (A/C): active and chronic lesions<br>IV (C): chronic lesions |
| Class V | Membranous lupus nephritis[c] |
| Class VI | Advanced sclerosing lupus nephritis (≥90% globally sclerosed glomeruli without residual activity) |

[a]Indicate the proportion of glomeruli with active and with sclerotic lesions
[b]Subclasses indicate the proportion of glomeruli with segmental or global disease, active and sclerotic lesions, fibrinoid necrosis, and cellular crescents. Subclasses may also indicate and grade (mild, moderate, severe) tubular atrophy, interstitial inflammation and fibrosis, severity of arteriosclerosis or other vascular lesions
[c]Class V may occur in combination with III or IV in which case both will be diagnosed

miscommunication and placing appropriate emphasis on the proliferative lesion
○ Additionally, sclerotic glomeruli representing chronic lupus nephritis must be considered when determining class
○ Class IV was divided into two subcategories based on whether the endocapillary involvement is predominantly segmental (class IV-S) or global (class IV-G)

## American College of Rheumatology guidelines for screening, treatment, and management of lupus nephritis

• Guidelines and recommendations developed and/or endorsed by the American College of Rheumatology (ACR) are intended to provide guidance for particular patterns of practice and not to dictate the care of a particular patient

- The ACR considers adherence to these guidelines and recommendations to be voluntary, with the ultimate determination regarding their application to be made by the physician in light of each patient's individual circumstances
- Guidelines and recommendations are intended to promote beneficial or desirable outcomes but cannot guarantee any specific outcome
- Guidelines have inherent limitations in informing individual patient care
  - Though they should not supplant clinical judgment or limit clinical judgment, they do provide expert advice to the practicing physician managing patient with lupus nephritis
- Guidelines and recommendations developed or endorsed by the ACR are subject to periodic revision as warranted by the evolution of medical knowledge, technology, and practice
- The guidelines apply to LN in adults, particularly to those receiving care in the US and include interventions that were available in the US as of February 2012
- The strength of the evidence was graded using methodology previously reported by the American College of Cardiology
  - Level A evidence represents data derived from multiple randomized clinical trials (RCTs) or a meta-analysis
  - Level B evidence represents data from a single randomized clinical trial or non-randomized study
  - Level C evidence represents data from consensus, expert opinion, or case series

## Case definition for LN

- LN is defined as clinical and laboratory manifestations that meet ACR criteria
  - Persistent proteinuria >0.5 g per day or >3+ protein on urine dipstick and/or cellular casts including red blood cells (RBCs), hemoglobin, granular, tubular, or mixed
- Spot urine protein/creatinine ratio of >0.5 can be substituted for the 24-hour protein measurement, and "active urinary sediment" (>5 RBCs/high-power field (hpf), >5 white blood cells (WBCs)/hpf in the absence of infection, or cellular casts limited to RBC or WBC casts) can be substituted for cellular casts
- Ideally, a renal biopsy consistent with an immune complex-mediated glomerulonephritis compatible with LN should be sought

## Renal biopsy and histology

> All patients with clinical evidence of active LN, previously untreated, should undergo renal biopsy (unless strongly contraindicated) so that glomerular disease can be classified by current ISN/RPS classification (level C evidence). This allows for evaluation for activity and chronicity and for tubular and vascular changes.

- Indications for renal biopsy in patients with SLE (all level C evidence):
  - Increasing serum creatinine without alternative causes
  - Proteinuria $\geq 1\,g/24$ hours
  - Any of the following combinations that are confirmed on at least two occasions within a short period of time and in the absence of other causes
    - Proteinuria $\geq 0.5\,g/24$ hours plus hematuria, defined as $\geq 5$ RBCs/hpf
    - Proteinuria $\geq 0.5\,g/24$ hours plus cellular casts

### Management
- Class I (minimal mesangial immune deposits on immunofluorescence with normal light microscopy) and class II (mesangial hypercellularity or matrix expansion on light microscopy with immune deposits confined to mesangium on immunofluorescence) generally do not require immunosuppressive treatment (level C evidence)
- In general, class III (subendothelial immune deposits with proliferative changes in <50% of glomeruli) and class IV (subendothelial deposits and proliferative glomerular changes involving ≥50% of glomeruli) require aggressive therapy with glucocorticoids and immunosuppressive agents
- Class V (subepithelial immune deposits and membranous thickening of glomerular capillaries), when combined with class III or IV should be treated in the same manner as class III or IV
- Class V alone (pure membranous LN) typically warrants immunosuppressive treatment when accompanied by nephrotic syndrome or an elevated or rising creatinine
- Class VI (sclerosis of ≥90% of glomeruli) generally indicates impending end-stage renal disease with little effect of immunosuppression

### Adjunctive treatments
- All SLE patients with LN should be treated with hydroxychloroquine (HCQ), unless a contraindication exists (level C evidence)
  - ○ HCQ reduces flare rates of lupus, lowers damage accrual, including renal damage, and may reduce risk of thrombotic events
- All LN with proteinuria ≥0.5 g/24 hours (or equivalent by spot urine ratios) should be treated with either angiotensin-converting enzyme (ACE) inhibitors or angiotensin receptor blockers (ARBs)
  - ○ These medications are contraindicated in pregnancy
- Hypertension should be strictly controlled, with a target of ≤130/80 mmHg (level A evidence)
- Statin therapy should be given in those with low-density lipoprotein cholesterol >100 mg/dL (level C evidence)

### Recommendations for induction treatments in those with ISN class III/IV LN
- Recommended treatment includes **mycophenolate mofetil (MMF)** at 2–3 g total daily orally or intravenous (IV) **cyclophosphamide (CYC)** along with glucocorticoids (level A evidence)
- Studies have shown MMF and CYC are considered equivalent in efficacy, though there is less long-term outcome data with MMF
  - ○ MMF has had similar efficacy in all races studies to date but MMF may be more likely to induce improvement in those who are African-American or Hispanic
  - ○ The ACR Task Force Panel voted that Asians compared to non-Asians might require lower doses of MMF for similar efficacy (level C evidence)
    - ▪ Asians might require a target of 2 g/day compared to 3 g in other racial/ethnic groups
- More severe LN, those with crescents and a recent significant rise in creatinine, should target 3 g of MMF per day
  - ○ Gastrointestinal (GI) symptoms, such as diarrhea and nausea, occur more frequently at higher doses
  - ○ Some evidence suggests that mycophenolic acid (MPA) and enteric-coated mycophenolate sodium are less likely than MMF to cause GI upset, though this is controversial and further studies using these preparations are in progress
- The Core Expert Panel recommended that MMF and MPA are equally likely to induce improvement of LN, with 1440–2160 mg total daily dose of MPA roughly equivalent to 2000–3000 mg total daily dose of MMF
- There is not enough data to make recommendations for monitoring serum levels of MPA, the active metabolite of MMF

- Two regimens of IV CYC are recommended:
  - **Low-dose "Euro-Lupus" CYC** (500 mg IV once every 2 weeks for a total of six doses), followed by maintenance therapy with daily oral azathioprine (AZA) or daily oral MMF (level B evidence)
    - Recommended for white patients with western European or southern European racial/ethnic backgrounds (level B evidence)
  - **High-dose "National Institutes of Health" CYC** (500–1000 mg/m$^2$ IV once a month for six doses), followed by maintenance treatment with MMF or AZA (level A evidence)
- Pulse IV glucocorticoids (500–1000 mg methylprednisolone daily for three doses) in combination with immunosuppressive therapy was recommended by the ACR Task Force Panel, followed by daily oral glucocorticoids (0.5–1 mg/kg/day), followed by a taper to the minimal amount necessary to control disease (level C evidence)
  - This recommendation was based primarily on consensus expert opinion with some recent trials employing pulse steroids at onset of treatment, compared to others which have not
  - There are insufficient data to recommend a specific steroid taper due to the variability of nephritis and extrarenal manifestations
- No consensus was reached regarding the use of monthly IV methylprednisolone with monthly IV CYC, though one study suggested benefit over IV CYC alone
- The panel recommended that most patients continue on either CYC or MMF for 6 months after initiation of induction before making major changes in treatment other than with glucocorticoids
  - The exception would be in the case of clear worsening at 3 months evidenced by 50% or more worsening of proteinuria or serum creatinine (level A evidence)
- MMF was preferred to CYC for patients who value preservation of fertility in both women and men (level A evidence)
  - The ACR Task Force Panel did not reach a consensus on the use of leuprolide as a means of preserving fertility in women
- MMF should not be used in anyone who is pregnant or is contemplating pregnancy (teratogenic, class D) and should be stopped for at least 6 weeks prior to conceiving

### Recommendations for induction of improvement in patients with class IV or IV/V plus cellular crescents

- **CYC** or **MMF** was recommended for this type of LN (level C evidence), along with IV pulses of high-dose glucocorticoid and initiation of oral glucocorticoids at 1 mg/kg/day

• The presence of any crescents on a renal biopsy sample was considered crescentic LN

## Recommendations for induction of improvement in patients with class V LN

• Pure membranous or class V LN with nephrotic range proteinuria should be started on prednisone (0.5 mg/kg/day) plus MMF 2–3 g total daily dose (level A evidence)
• There was no consensus on other therapies that have been reported

## Recommendations for maintaining improvement in patients who respond to induction therapy

• AZA or MMF should be used for maintenance therapy (level A evidence)
• There are no data to date that show how rapidly AZA or MMF can be tapered or withdrawn

## Recommendations for changing therapies in patients who do not respond adequately to induction therapy

• If after 6 months of glucocorticoids plus MMF or CYC, a patient fails treatment based on the treating physician's clinical impression, the immunosuppressive agent should be switched from either CYC to MMF, or from MMF to CYC, with these changes accompanied by IV pulses of glucocorticoids for 3 days (level C evidence)
   ○ In white individuals, the CYC can be either low or high dose, though evidence to support this is not as strong as for initial induction therapy
• In some cases, rituximab can be used in patients whose nephritis fails to improve or worsen after 6 months of one induction therapy or after failing both CYC and MMF (level C evidence)
• Though evidence exists for their efficacy as an induction agent and in refractory disease, consensus was not reached regarding the use of calcineurin inhibitors in this setting
• If nephritis is worsening after 3 months of glucocorticoids plus CYC or MMF, any of the alternative treatments discussed can be used (level C evidence)
   ○ There is not enough evidence to support certain combinations that are being studied, such as MMF and calcineurin inhibitors or rituximab and MMF
   ○ Belimumab (anti-BLyS/BAFF), approved for non-renal active lupus, is currently being studied in LN

## Vascular involvement in SLE with renal abnormalities
- Renal tissue can exhibit a variety of vascular involvement
  - Vasculitis
  - Fibrinoid necrosis with narrowing of small arteries/arterioles ("bland" vasculopathy – associated with hypertension)
  - Thrombotic microangiopathy
  - Renal vein thrombosis
- The Task Force Panel recommended that thrombotic microangiopathy be treated primarily with plasma exchange therapy (level C evidence)

## Treatment of LN in patients who are pregnant
- All approaches in this section are level C evidence
- Those with prior LN but no current evidence of activity do not require treatment
- Those with mild systemic activity may be treated with HCQ
- If clinically active nephritis is present or substantial extrarenal activity, glucocorticoids may be used at doses necessary to control disease activity
  - This is associated with higher risks for hypertension and diabetes mellitus
- AZA can be added if necessary and should not exceed 2mg/kg in pregnant women
  - Although AZA is listed as pregnancy category D, studies have shown that the risk of fetal abnormalities is low
- MMF, CYC, and methotrexate must be avoided due to their teratogencity
- Consideration should be given to deliver after 28 weeks, or the earliest period in which it is felt a viable fetus can be delivered, in those with persistently active LN with documented or suspected class III or IV with crescents

## Monitoring activity of LN
- LN activity may be monitored by regular physician visits in which blood pressure, urinalysis, protein/creatinine ratio, serum creatinine, C3/C4 levels, and anti-DNA antibodies are assessed
- The frequency of monitoring depends on the activity of nephritis at the onset of treatment
  - Patients with active nephritis should have blood pressure and renal studies every month, with C3/C4 and anti-DNA antibodies assessed every 2–3 months

○ Pregnant patients with active LN should be assessed with a similar program, but with C3/C4 and anti-DNA antibodies assessed monthly as well

○ Patients with a history of prior active LN should be monitored every 3 months

○ Pregnant patients with a history of prior active LN should be assessed with a similar program, but with blood pressure and urinalysis screening monthly during pregnancy

○ Patients without a history of prior or current LN should have their blood pressure checked every 3 months, with the remaining assessments at least every 6 months

## Further reading

Canadian Hydroxychloroquine Study Group (1991) A randomized study of the effect of withdrawing hydroxychloroquine sulfate in systemic lupus erythematosus. *The New England Journal of Medicine* 324(3): 150–154.

Contreras, G., Pardo, V., Leclercq, B., et al. (2004) Sequential therapies for proliferative lupus nephritis. *The New England Journal of Medicine* 350(10): 971–980.

Fessler, B.J., Alarcon, G.S., McGwin, G., Jr., et al. (2005) Systemic lupus erythematosus in three ethnic groups: XVI. Association of hydroxychloroquine use with reduced risk of damage accrual. *Arthritis and Rheumatism* 52(5): 1473–1480.

Furie, R., Petrie, M., Zamani, O., et al. (2011) A phase III, randomized, placebo-controlled study of belimumab, a monoclonal antibody that inhibits B lymphocyte stimulator, in patients with systemic lupus erythematosus. *Arthritis and Rheumatism* 63(12): 3918–3930.

Hahn, B.H., McMahon, M.A., Wilkinson, A., et al. (2012) American College of Rheumatology guidelines for screening, treatment, and management of lupus nephritis. *Arthritis Care & Research* 64(6): 797–808.

Houssiau, F.A., Vasconcelos, C., D'Cruz, D., et al. (2010) The 10-year follow-up data of the Euro-Lupus Nephritis Trial comparing low-dose and high-dose intravenous cyclophosphamide. *Annals of Rheumatic Disease* 69(1): 61–64.

Houssiau, F.A., Vasconcelos, C., D'Cruz, D., et al. (2002) Immunosuppressive therapy in lupus nephritis: the Euro-Lupus Nephritis Trial, a randomized trial of low-dose versus high-dose intravenous cyclophosphamide. *Arthritis and Rheumatism* 46(8): 2121–2131.

Hunt, S.A. (2005) ACC/AHA 2005 guideline update for the diagnosis and management of chronic heart failure in the adult: a report of the American College of Cardiology/American Heart Association Task Force on Practice Guidelines (Writing Committee to Update the 2001 Guidelines for the Evaluation and Management of Heart Failure). *Journal of the American College of Cardiology* 46(6): e1–82.

Jung, H., Bobba, R., Su, J., et al. (2010) The protective effect of antimalarial drugs on thrombovascular events in systemic lupus erythematosus. *Arthritis and Rheumatism* 62(3): 863–868.

Merrill, J.T., Neuwelt, C.M., Wallace, D.J., et al. (2010) Efficacy and safety of rituximab in moderately-to-severely active systemic lupus erythematosus: the randomized, double-blind, phase II/III systemic lupus erythematosus evaluation of rituximab trial. *Arthritis and Rheumatism* 62(1): 222–233.

Navarra, S.V., Guzman, R.M., Gallacher, A.E., et al. (2011) Efficacy and safety of belimumab in patients with active systemic lupus erythematosus: a randomised, placebo-controlled, phase 3 trial. *Lancet* 377(9767): 721–731.

Rovin, B.H., Furie, R., Latinis, K., et al. (2012) Efficacy and safety of rituximab in patients with active proliferative lupus nephritis: the Lupus Nephritis Assessment with Rituximab study. *Arthritis and Rheumatism* 64(4): 1215–1226.

Sanz, I., Lee, F.E. (2010) B cells as therapeutic targets in SLE. *Nature Reviews Rheumatology* 6(6): 326–337.

Ward, M.M., Pyun, E., Studenski, S. (1996) Mortality risks associated with specific clinical manifestations of systemic lupus erythematosus. *Archives of Internal Medicine* 156(12): 1337–1344.

Weening, J.J., D'Agati, V.D., Schwartz, M.M., et al. (2004) The classification of glomerulonephritis in systemic lupus erythematosus revisited. *Kidney International* 65(2): 521–530.

Weening, J.J., D'Agati, V.D., Schwartz, M.M., et al. (2004) The classification of glomerulonephritis in systemic lupus erythematosus revisited. *Journal of the American Society of Nephrology* 15(2): 241–250.

# CHAPTER 4

# Antiphospholipid antibody syndrome

**Cristina Drenkard**

Emory University School of Medicine, Atlanta, GA, USA

## Introduction

Antiphospholipid antibody syndrome (APS) is an autoimmune prothrombotic disorder characterized by the occurrence of venous or arterial thrombosis or pregnancy morbidity and the persistent presence of antiphospholipid antibodies.

• APS may present associated with other autoimmune diseases (more frequently SLE) or as a primary condition (PAPS)

• Antiphospholipid antibodies (aPL) are a family of antibodies directed against phospholipid–protein complexes, which include lupus anticoagulant (LAC), anticardiolipin antibodies (aCL), and anti-beta-2 glycoprotein I (anti-β2GPI) antibodies

• aPL have been shown to target a number of phospholipid-binding proteins such as prothrombin, though it is generally accepted that aPL targeting the plasma protein β2-glycoprotein I (β2GPI) are the most relevant

## Epidemiology

• There are no population-based studies on the prevalence of APL syndrome

*Rheumatology Board Review*, First Edition. Edited by Karen Law and Aliza Lipson.

- The prevalence of aPL antibodies ranges from 1–10% in the general population (usually transient low-titer aCL, with the elderly at the higher end of the range)
- The strength of association between aPL and thrombosis varies among studies depending on the aPL test type, transient versus persistent positive aPL, study design, and clinical populations studied
- Limited number of uncontrolled and non risk-stratified studies show that individuals with no history of vascular or pregnancy events who are aPL-positive have 0–4% risk of annual thrombosis
- Persistent positive titers of aPL and presence of three types of aPL (triple positive) increase the risk of thrombosis
- Approximately 5–20% of patients presenting with thrombosis have aPL
- aPL antibodies are present in 16% of patients with rheumatoid arthritis, and in 30–40% of patients with SLE
- Patients with other autoimmune diseases such as SLE have increased risk of thrombotic or obstetric clinical manifestations associated with aPL

## Classification criteria

According to the Revised Sapporo Classification Criteria for the Antiphospholipid Syndrome, **APS is present if at least one of the clinical criteria and one of the laboratory criteria (listed below) are met**:

### Clinical criteria
- **Vascular thrombosis**
  - One or more clinical episodes of arterial, venous, or small vessel thrombosis, in any tissue or organ
- **Pregnancy morbidity**
  - One or more unexplained deaths of a morphologically normal fetus at or beyond the 10th week of gestation, or
  - One or more premature births of a morphologically normal neonate before the 34th week of gestation because of eclampsia, severe preeclampsia, or recognized features of placental insufficiency, or
  - Three or more unexplained consecutive spontaneous abortions before the 10th week of gestation, with maternal anatomic or hormonal abnormalities and paternal and maternal chromosomal causes excluded

### Laboratory criteria
- **Lupus anticoagulant** present in plasma, on two or more occasions at least 12 weeks apart, detected according to the guidelines of the International Society on Thrombosis and Hemostasis

• **Anticardiolipin antibody of IgG and/or IgM isotype** in serum or plasma, present in medium or high titer (i.e. >40 GPL or MPL, or greater than the 99th percentile), on two or more occasions, at least 12 weeks apart, measured by a standardized enzyme-linked immunosorbent assay (ELISA)

• **Anti-β2-glycoprotein I antibody of IgG and/or IgM isotype** in serum or plasma (in titer greater than the 99th percentile) present on two or more occasions, at least 12 weeks apart, measured by a standardized ELISA

## Important considerations stated by the revised Sapporo classification criteria for the APS

• When less than 12 weeks or more than 5 years separate the positive aPL test and the clinical manifestation, classification of APS should be avoided

• Patients should not be excluded from APS trials if coexisting inherited or acquired factors for thrombosis are present

• Presence and absence of additional risk factors for thrombosis should be recognized to further classify APS patients

• Investigators involved in population studies are advised to classify APS patients into four different categories of aPL assay positivity (see Miyakis et al. 2006)

## The clinical spectrum of APS

• The clinical spectrum of patients with positive aPL is widely heterogeneous, including different subgroups:
  ○ Antiphospholipid syndrome with vascular events
  ○ Antiphospholipid syndrome with only pregnancy morbidity
  ○ Antiphospholipid syndrome with both vascular and pregnancy morbidity
  ○ Non-criteria aPL manifestations
    ▪ Skin ulcers
    ▪ Livedo reticularis
    ▪ Thrombocytopenia
    ▪ Hemolytic anemia
    ▪ Antiphospholipid antibody nephropathy
    ▪ Cardiac valve disease
    ▪ Chorea
    ▪ Cognitive dysfunction
    ▪ Diffuse alveolar hemorrhage

○ Catastrophic antiphospholipid syndrome
○ Asymptomatic aPL positivity

## aPL antibodies laboratory testing

### Lupus anticoagulants (LACs)
• LACs prolong phospholipid-dependent coagulation tests due to antagonism of reagent phospholipids
• No single test will identify all LACs, and it is recommended to perform at least two screening assays
• The risk of false-positive results may be increased to an unacceptable level if more than two screening tests are performed
• The most commonly used screening assays include the activated partial thromboplastin time (APTT) and dilute Russell viper venom time (DRVVT)
• The prothrombin time is not usually prolonged because of the large amount of phospholipid in the thromboplastin reagent
• The results of screening tests are considered suggestive of LAC when clotting times are longer than the local cut-off value
• A positive screen is followed by a mixing study
  ○ Lupus anticoagulants demonstrate an inhibitor pattern in mixing studies wherein the prolonged coagulation time fails to correct by mixing patient and pooled normal plasma
• The presence of LAC is confirmed by demonstrating shortening of the prolonged coagulation time on addition of excess phospholipids

### aCL antibodies and anti-β2GPI antibodies
• Testing for aCL and anti-β2GPI antibodies (IgG and IgM) by ELISA should be performed concurrently with LAC testing if APS is suspected
• Anticardiolipin results are considered positive if present in moderate to high titer, whereas anti-β2GPI results are positive in titer greater than the 99th percentile
• Cardiolipin is a negatively charged phospholipid, and aCL antibodies in APS typically require a protein cofactor (such as β2GPI) to create the antigenic target (phospholipid–protein complex)
  ○ Transient aCL antibodies have been identified during infections which characteristically do not have a reactivity against β2GPI
  ○ Therefore, β2GPI-dependent aCL assays are recommended
• In general, the aCL assay is more sensitive for APS, whereas the β2GPI assay is more specific

## Limitations of aPL testing

- Classification criteria for definite antiphospholipid syndrome require a positive laboratory test between one or more of the three types of assays used to detect aPL (aCL IgG and IgM, anti-β2GPI antibodies IgG and IgM, and/or LAC)
- The clinical and diagnostic value of aPL tests is limited by significant interassay and interlaboratory variation in the results of LAC, aCL and anti-β2GPI assays
- High variability in the sensitivity and specificity of the tests is observed
- Major limitations on clinical aPL testing are related to
  - Lack of broad international consensus guidelines on the recommended best practices for testing LAC, aCL, and anti-β2GPI antibodies
  - Lack of laboratory standardization in units of measurement
  - Inconsistent calibration curves
  - Non-standardized cut-off values

The wide variability in the specificity and predictive value of the aPL antibodies is a longstanding problem related to poor standardization of aPL antibodies. In order to make clinical studies of patients with APS more comparable, the updated Sapporo Criteria introduced the concept of subclassification according to a single positive aPL test result or positive results of multiple aPL tests. Additionally, in 2010 an International Task Force of researchers and scientific experts in the field developed consensus guidelines on the recommended best practices for clinical labs, manufacturers, and research labs on immunoassays of LAC, aCL, and anti-β2GPI antibodies. In addition to technical recommendations, the Task Force recommended that labs report the results in units and in semi-quantitative ranges. The Task Force strongly recommended that labs include comments to assist clinicians in the interpretation of test results, and manufacturers disclose information based on evidence derived from clinical studies that may assist clinicians with the interpretation of results.

## Who should be tested?

- Laboratory testing should be limited to patients who have a significant probability of having APS
- The International Society on Thrombosis and Haemostasis subcommittee recommends categorizing patients according to clinical characteristics

into low, moderate, and high priority for LAC testing to minimize the risk of a false-positive result

- ○ **Low risk**: venous or arterial thromboembolism in elderly patients
- ○ **Moderate risk**: accidentally found prolonged APTT in asymptomatic subjects, recurrent spontaneous early pregnancy loss, unprovoked venous thromboembolism in young patients
- ○ **High risk**: unprovoked venous thromboembolism and unexplained arterial thrombosis in young patients (<50 years), thrombosis at unusual sites, late pregnancy loss, any thrombosis or pregnancy morbidity in patients with autoimmune diseases (SLE, rheumatoid arthritis, autoimmune thrombocytopenia, autoimmune hemolytic anemia)
- **Any positive laboratory test needs to be repeated 12 or more weeks following the initial positive laboratory result**
  - ○ This helps to exclude transient APAs, which are often secondary to intercurrent infection or other acute illness

## Who should not be tested?

- Testing asymptomatic individuals or categories of patients other than described above is highly discouraged to avoid the risk of obtaining false-positive results that are relatively common because of the poor specificity of the assays

## Testing individuals on anticoagulant therapy

- Anticoagulant medications such as heparin, direct thrombin inhibitors, and vitamin K antagonists (warfarin) can interfere with LAC testing due to their effects on coagulation assays
- Heparin and direct thrombin inhibitors are of particular concern because they prolong phospholipid-dependent coagulation tests and behave as inhibitors in mixing studies, potentially mimicking an LAC
- A thrombin time, or other means of identifying heparin, should be routinely performed on test plasma to identify the presence of heparin or direct thrombin inhibitors
- The commercial DRVVT reagents used for LAC testing contain heparin neutralizers; however, if the content of heparin in the test plasma exceeds the reagent neutralization capacity (typically greater than 0.8–1.0 U/mL), it can give rise to a false-positive LAC test result
- APTT reagents generally do not neutralize heparin
- Low-molecular weight heparin has less effect on LAC testing than unfractionated heparin
- In general, blood for LAC testing should be collected before starting anticoagulant drugs or after their discontinuation

- For vitamin K antagonists, wait 1–2 weeks after discontinuation or until the international normalized ratio (INR) is less than 1.5

## Treatment

### Primary and secondary prevention of thrombosis in individuals with aPL

- Current recommendations on the primary and secondary thrombo-prophylaxis in individuals with aPL are based on a consensus document elaborated after a systematic and critical review of the literature by an International Task Force composed of clinicians and researchers with experience in the field (in the setting of the 13th International Congress on Antiphospholipid Antibodies, held in Galveston in April 2010)
- High and low risk serological criteria are taken into consideration to manage APS patients
  - **High risk**
    - LAC positivity
    - Triple positivity (LAC + aCL + anti-β2GPI)
    - Isolated persistently positive aCL at medium–high titers
  - **Low risk**
    - Isolated, intermittently positive aCL or anti-β2GPI at low–medium titers
- The strength of the recommendations and the level of evidence were rated from 1–2 and from A–C, respectively, using the American College of Chest Physicians system
- Most of these recommendations are based on weak or incomplete data (evidence level C)

### General measures for aPL carriers

- A strict control of cardiovascular risk factors in all individuals with a high-risk aPL profile, irrespective of the presence of previous thrombosis, concomitant SLE or additional APS features (non-graded recommendation)
- All aPL carriers should receive thromboprophylaxis with usual doses of low molecular weight heparin in high-risk situations, such as surgery, prolonged immobilization, and the puerperium (1C recommendation)

### Primary thromboprophylaxis in SLE patients with aPL

- Clinicians should regularly assess patients with SLE for the presence of aPL (non-graded recommendation)

• Patients with SLE and positive LAC or isolated persistent aCL at medium–high titers should receive primary thromboprophylaxis with hydroxychloroquine (1B–2B recommendation) and low-dose aspirin (2B recommendation)

## Primary thromboprophylaxis in aPL-positive individuals with no previous thrombosis and without SLE

• Long-term thromboprophylaxis with low-dose aspirin in those with a high-risk aPL profile, especially in the presence of other thrombotic risk factors (2C recommendation)

## Secondary thromboprophylaxis

• Patients with either arterial or venous thrombosis and aPL who do not fulfill criteria for APS should be managed in the same manner as aPL-negative patients with similar thrombotic events (1C recommendation)
• Patients with definite APS and a first venous event should receive oral anticoagulant therapy to a target INR 2.0–3.0 (1B recommendation)
• Patients with definite APS and arterial thrombosis should be treated with warfarin at an INR >3.0 or combined antiaggregant–anticoagulant (INR 2.0–3.0) therapy (non-graded recommendation due to lack of consensus)
  ○ Some members of the Task Force believe that other options such as antiaggregant therapy alone or anticoagulant therapy to a target INR 2.0–3.0 would be equally valid in this setting
• An estimation of the patient's bleeding risk should be performed before prescribing high-intensity anticoagulant or combined antiaggregant–anticoagulant therapy (non-graded recommendation)
• Non-SLE patients with a first non-cardioembolic cerebral arterial event, with a low-risk aPL profile and the presence of reversible trigger factors, could individually be considered candidates for treatment with antiplatelet agents (non-graded recommendation)

## Duration of treatment

• Indefinite antithrombotic therapy in patients with definite APS and thrombosis (1C recommendation)
• In cases of first venous event, low-risk aPL profile, and a known transient precipitating factor, anticoagulation could be limited to 3–6 months (non-graded recommendation)

## Refractory and difficult cases

• In patients with difficult management due to recurrent thrombosis, fluctuating INR levels, major bleeding or a high risk for major bleeding, alternative therapies could include long-term low molecular weight heparin, hydroxychloroquine or statins (non-graded recommendation)

## Management of pregnancy outcomes in women with aPL

- The current standard of care for the prevention of fetal loss in patients diagnosed with APS is based on a low level of evidence because of the limited number of well designed controlled studies
- A meta-analysis of randomized–controlled trials and meta-regression concluded that the combination of heparin and aspirin is superior to aspirin alone in achieving more live births in patients with positive aPL antibodies and recurrent pregnancy loss
- Prophylactic dose heparin (e.g. enoxaparin 30–40 mg SC once daily) is used for patients with APS fulfilling the Sapporo Criteria based on a history of pregnancy morbidity only
- Therapeutic dose heparin (e.g. enoxaparin 1 mg/kg SC twice daily or 1.5 mg/kg SC once daily) is used for patients with APS fulfilling the Sapporo Criteria based on a thrombotic vascular event regardless of pregnancy history
- Low-dose aspirin for asymptomatic (no history of vascular or pregnancy events) significantly aPL-positive patients is generally used during pregnancy (no data support this strategy)
- The postpartum period carries a high risk of maternal thrombosis, especially in patients with history of thrombosis and/or those undergoing cesarean deliveries
  - Patients who have had thrombotic events and had been using warfarin should be restarted on warfarin after the delivery
  - Patients who have had pregnancy events only should be continued on heparin for 8–12 weeks

## Further reading

Barbhaiya, M., Erkan, D. (2011) Primary thrombosis prophylaxis in antiphospholipid antibody-positive patients: where do we stand? *Current Rheumatology Reports* 13(1): 59–69.

Erkan D., Lockshin, M.D. (2010) Non-criteria manifestations of antiphospholipid syndrome. *Lupus* 19: 424–427.

George, D., Erkan, D. (2009) Antiphospholipid syndrome. *Progress in Cardiovascular Diseases* 52(2): 115–125.

Lakos, G., Favaloro, E.J., Harris, E.N., et al. (2012) International consensus guidelines on anticardiolipin and anti-beta2-glycoprotein I testing: report from the 13th International Congress on Antiphospholipid Antibodies. *Arthritis and Rheumatism* 64(1): 1–10.

Mak, A., Cheung, M.-W.L., Cheak, A.A., et al. (2010) Combination of heparin and aspirin is superior to aspirin alone in enhancing live births in patients with recurrent pregnancy loss and positive anti-phospholipid antibodies: a meta-analysis of randomized controlled trials and meta-regression. *Rheumatology (Oxford)* 49(2): 281–288.

Miyakis, S., Lockshin, M.D., Atsumi, T., et al. (2006) International consensus statement on an update of the classification criteria for definite antiphospholipid syndrome (APS). *Journal of Thrombosis and Haemostasis* 4(2): 295–306.

Pengo, V., Tripodi, A., Reber, G., et al. (2009) Update of the guidelines for lupus anti-coagulant detection. Subcommittee on Lupus Anticoagulant/Antiphospholipid Antibody of the Scientific and Standardisation Committee of the International Society on Thrombosis and Haemostasis. *Journal of Thrombosis and Haemostasis* 7(10): 1737–1740.

Pierangeli, S.S., Favaloro, E.J., Lakos, G., et al. (2012) Standards and reference materials for the anticardiolipin and anti-beta2glycoprotein I assays: a report of recommendations from the APL Task Force at the 13th International Congress on Antiphospholipid Antibodies. *Clinica Chimica Acta* 413(1-2): 358–360.

Ruiz-Irastorza, G., Cuadrado, M.J., Ruiz-Arruza, I., et al. (2011) Evidence-based recommendations for the prevention and long-term management of thrombosis in antiphospholipid antibody-positive patients: report of a task force at the 13th International Congress on antiphospholipid antibodies. *Lupus* 20(2): 206–218.

## CHAPTER 5

# IgG4-related disease

## Arezou Khosroshahi

Emory University School of Medicine, Atlanta, GA, USA

## Introduction

IgG4-related disease (IgG4-RD) is a systemic fibro-inflammatory condition formally recognized as an entity in the past decade. This condition is defined by its highly characteristic histopathology and immunostaining pattern that is similar across the organ systems involved. Regardless of the affected organ, these patients share **unique clinical features** including:

- tendency to form **mass lesions**;
- **elevated serum IgG4** concentration (in the majority of patients);
- excellent **response to glucocorticoid treatment**.

This disease was first identified in the pancreas as "autoimmune pancreatitis" (AIP). In 2001, AIP was linked to elevated serum IgG4 concentrations, and shortly thereafter, to the presence of large numbers of IgG4-positive plasma cells in the pancreatic tissues. A variety of extrapancreatic lesions was observed to occur in patients with AIP that shared the same pathological features found in the pancreas. This observation led to the proposal of a new systemic condition now called IgG4-related disease (IgG4-RD).

> IgG4-RD is now known to involve almost any organ system, including pancreas, liver, salivary glands, periorbital tissues (e.g. the lacrimal gland and retro-orbital space), lungs, aorta, kidneys, lymph nodes, retroperitoneum, meninges, thyroid gland, pericardium, prostate, and skin.

---

*Rheumatology Board Review*, First Edition. Edited by Karen Law and Aliza Lipson.
© 2014 John Wiley & Sons, Inc. Published 2014 by John Wiley & Sons, Inc.

Multiple organ involvement can occur simultaneously; it may also precede or develop years after the initial recognition of the index organ.

Although it is not clear if autoimmunity plays any role in the etiology of this condition, rheumatology is probably the most appropriate specialty to manage this disease for several reasons:

- it is an immune-mediated fibrosing condition;
- it mimics other systemic rheumatologic conditions;
- it responds well to steroid treatment.

Additionally, many known entities followed by rheumatologists are now recognized to be part of the IgG4-RD spectrum, including Mikulicz's disease, retroperitoneal fibrosis, multifocal fibrosclerosis, lymphoplasmacytic aortitis, and inflammatory orbital pseudotumors.

## Histology

- Two distinct features link separate manifestations of IgG4-RD in different organs and unify variable entities as one systemic condition
  - ○ A unique histopathologic appearance
  - ○ **Abundance of IgG4+ plasma cells** in the tissue (Figure 5.1)

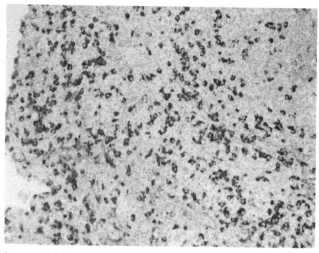

**Figure 5.1** Immunostaining for IgG4 in IgG4-RD. The majority of plasma cells appear positive for IgG4 (Color plate 5.1).

The major characteristic histologic features of IgG4-RD are:
- Dense lymphoplasmacytic infiltrate rich in IgG4+ plasma cells
- Storiform pattern of fibrosis
- Obliterative phlebitis

- **Modest eosinophilia** in the tissue is also a common finding
- Fibrosis in IgG4-RD is mostly organized, at least focally, in a storiform pattern (Figure 5.2)
  - ○ The storiform pattern resembles the spokes of a cartwheel with spindle cells radiating from the center

Features that are **inconsistent** with the diagnosis of IgG4-RD are the presence of granulomas and prominent neutrophilic infiltrate. Giant cells, neutrophilic microabscesses, and areas of necrosis are not usually seen in this condition.

- Initially, increased number of IgG4+ plasma cells was the hallmark of the disease
  - ○ As knowledge with regard to this condition grew it was realized that the abundance of IgG4+ plasma cells in the absence of

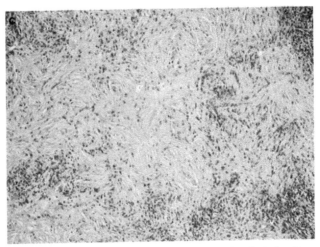

**Figure 5.2** IgG4-related disease typically shows an irregularly whorled pattern of fibrosis (storiform fibrosis) associated with lymphoplasmacytic infiltration (Color plate 5.2).

compatible specific histology could be found in a wide spectrum of diseases

○ **Abundance of IgG4+ plasma cells alone is not adequate as a distinguishing feature in IgG4-related disease**

## Epidemiology

• The overall epidemiology of IgG4-RD in the general population remains unknown

• This condition usually affects elderly men with a mean age between 58 and 69 years

• The male to female ratio is reported as 4:1, although studies of patients with only head and neck involvement of the disease show almost equal sex distributions

• IgG4-RD was initially recognized in Japan and most studies reported in the literature are from Japan

○ Knowledge has spread to investigators and clinicians around the world, and it seems that the disease occurs in every geographic and ethnic population with no obvious preference

○ Definitive assessment of its incidence and prevalence among all populations as a systemic disease requires multinational cohorts studying IgG4-RD, which are lacking at this point

## Etiology

• The pathogenesis of IgG4-RD is poorly understood

• Based on serological, immunological, and molecular studies it is suggested that autoimmunity, allergy (hypersensitivity), or molecular mimicry may play roles in its mechanism of disease

• The IgG4 molecule is postulated to be a protective antibody with regard to allergens and certain infectious agents like parasites

○ It typically appears after prolonged immunization, especially in the context of IgE-mediated allergy and immunotherapy, but its exact physiologic role is poorly understood

○ In the past decades, our understanding about the role of IgG4 in different immune-mediated conditions has changed remarkably

▪ IgG4 antibodies against desmoglein 1 play a major role in blister formation in pemphigus vulgaris and foliaceus

▪ IgG4 antibodies against M-type phospholipase A2 receptor cause idiopathic memebranous glomerulonephritis

▪ Antibodies against the metalloproteinase ADAMTS13, which is the pathogenic antibody in thrombotic thrombocytopenic purpura, are IgG4 antibodies

→ For these reasons, this molecule is not just an immune-modulating and anti-inflammatory antibody
- At the same time, the IgG4 molecule is present in the involved tissues with chronic inflammation in certain conditions like rheumatoid arthritis, granulomatosis with polyangiitis, and sarcoidosis
○ The role of IgG4 molecules in IgG4-RD is still uncertain
- No specific autoantigen has been identified, and it is not clear whether the IgG4 antibodies are a byproduct of certain types of inflammation or pathogenic themselves in this condition

## Clinical manifestations

- The initial presentation of patients with IgG4-RD is often a mass that has developed subacutely in the affected organ, causing symptoms due to mass effect or damage to the organ
  ○ Painless jaundice due to a mass or swelling in the head of the pancreas
  ○ Pseudotumor of the orbit
  ○ Pulmonary nodule resembling cancer
- Patients rarely manifest constitutional symptoms of fever or weight loss
- A history of asthma, eczema, or atopy is commonly reported
- Multiple organ involvement is reported in 60–90% of patients but may not all be symptomatic at diagnosis
- Forty percent of patients with IgG4-RD have lymphadenopathy at the time of their presentation
- Serum inflammatory markers such as the erythrocyte sedimentation rate (ESR) and C-reactive protein (CRP) are usually modestly elevated
- Increased levels of serum IgE and peripheral eosinophilia can be found in some patients
- Antinuclear antibody (ANA) assays are positive in more than half of all patients with IgG4-RD, but specific extractable nuclear antigen autoantibodies such as anti-Ro/SSA and La/SSB are absent
- IgG4-RD can involve almost any organ system
  ○ The relative frequency of different organ involvements are not accurately reported because most of the cohorts studying this condition were designed to study a certain organ-specific index illness
  ○ Based on one study looking at 114 patients with IgG4-RD in Japan, the most commonly affected organs are:
    - Liver and bile ducts (38%)
    - Salivary glands (34%)
    - Lung and pleura (26%)

- Pancreas (24%)
- Lacrimal glands (12%)
- Retroperitoneum (11%)
- Kidney (9%)
- Aorta (9%)
- Gallbladder (8%)

   o These frequencies may vary slightly in different studies but these organs are among the most commonly involved organs in IgG4-RD

## Differential diagnosis

• The differential diagnosis of IgG4-RD includes a wide range of rheumatic, infectious, and malignant conditions and depends on the specific organ involvement and clinical presentation

• Careful exclusion of malignancy in the specific organ system is critical in evaluation of these patients

• Lymphoproliferative disorders, especially **low-grade B cell lymphomas**, **granulomatosis with polyangiitis**, and **sarcoidosis** are among the leading mimics for IgG4-RD

## Specific organ involvement in IgG4-RD

### Head and neck area
### Salivary glands

• IgG4-related sialadenitis is probably the most common IgG4-RD manifestation evaluated by rheumatologists

• Many patients with this condition are erroneously diagnosed as having Sjögren's syndrome (SJS), with negative antibodies to Ro and La and good response to steroids

   o Swelling of the salivary gland is more prominent in IgG4-related siladenitis, while sicca symptoms are not as common unless patients have fibrotic, damaged organs due to longstanding disease

• Parotids, submandibular glands, and minor salivary glands can be affected in this condition

• Mikulicz disease, which was believed to be a variant of SJS and is defined by symmetric, bilateral, painless swelling of the submandibular, parotid, and lacrimal glands, is now proved to be IgG4-RD

• Chronic sclerosing sialadenitis, called Küttner's tumor, is another entity that is now recognized as IgG4-related sialadenitis in the absence of stones and infections

## Lacrimal glands and other ophthalmic involvement
• IgG4-related dacryoadenitis (involvement of the lacrimal gland) is the most common manifestation of the IgG4-RD in the orbital area
• Many other "idiopathic" orbital inflammations including pseudotumors of the orbit, orbital myositis, uveitis, iritis, and inflammation of optic nerve sheath have been discovered to be manifestations of IgG4-RD

## Thyroid
• IgG4-RD involvement of the thyroid manifests as Riedel's thyroiditis
• This condition has been part of the mutifocal fibrosclerosis syndrome, another IgG4-RD syndrome described centuries ago
• Prevalence of hypothyroidism has been reported to be high in patients with IgG4-RD but no definite relationship has been found between other thyroid conditions and IgG4-RD

## Meninges
• A recent study showed that 27% of idiopathic cases of pachymeningitis are IgG4-related pachymeningitis
• Patients usually present with radiculomyelopathy, headache, or cranial nerve palsies
• Exclusion of other causes of pachymeningitis, such as lymphoma, granulomatosis with polyangiitis, or sarcoidosis, requires thorough evaluation of a biopsy specimen

## Pituitary gland
• Hypophysitis associated with IgG4-RD has been reported which usually manifests with clinical pituitary insufficiency in the setting of pituitary mass
• Involvement of other organs with IgG4-RD and elevated serum IgG4 concentration are usually helpful for the diagnosis, otherwise exclusion of other infiltrative process including malignancy is required for appropriate management

## Peripheral nervous system
• IgG4-RD has not been reported as central nervous system involvement including brain or spinal cord paranchymal lesions
• As IgG4-RD patients continue to have more extensive imaging evaluations, reports of associated peripheral nerve lesions are increasing in frequency
• These peripheral nerve lesions present as perineural masses, primarily in the orbit or paravertebral areas

## Thoracic area

### Lungs

- Pulmonary involvement of IgG4-RD is one of the most common manifestations of this systemic condition
- Many patients are either asymptomatic or have chronic respiratory symptoms
- The workup reveals lung nodules, ground glass opacities, alveolar/interstitial inflammation, bronchovascular bundle thickening, or pleural thickening and effusion
- Large airway disease causing tracheobronchial stenosis has been reported in IgG4-RD

### Aorta

- IgG4-RD accounts for a significant proportion of inflammatory aortitis both in the thoracic and abdominal aorta
- Many cases described as chronic sclerosing aortitis or even isolated aortitis can be diagnosed as IgG4-RD with thorough evaluation
- IgG4-related aortitis is one of the most critical manifestations of IgG4-RD which requires immediate treatment to prevent fatal complications including ruptured aortic aneurysm (Figure 5.3)

### Pericardium

- Constrictive pericarditis with extensive fibrosis and abundant inflammation has been reported in association with IgG4-RD
- Pericardial thickening and effusions are findings that can be observed in imaging evaluations of patients with other organ involvements

## Abdomen and pelvic area

### Pancreas

- IgG4-RD was initially identified in the pancreas as autoimmune pancreatitis (AIP)
- This term now describes two different immune-mediated diseases in the pancreas
  - **AIP type 1** is the pancreatic involvement of the IgG4-RD which is defined by lymphoplasmacytic sclerosing pancreatitis
  - **AIP type 2**, characterized by granulocytic epithelial lesions, is not part of IgG4-RD
- Patients with type 1 AIP or IgG4-related pancreatitis usually present with painless jaundice, weight loss, and mild abdominal discomfort
- The classic radiologic findings in AIP include either a diffusely swollen, sausage-shaped pancreas or a localized mass

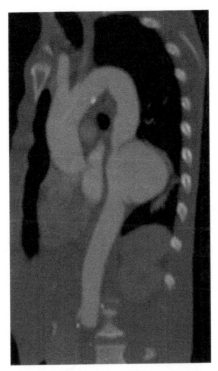

**Figure 5.3** Computed tomographic angiogram (CTA) imaging of aortic aneurysm in a patient with IgG4-related aortitis. It shows an expanding aneurysmal mass of the descending thoracic aorta.

 ○ These symptoms lead the clinician to suspect the diagnosis of pancreatic cancer rather than pancreatitis
 ○ For this reason, AIP is diagnosed many times in patients who have undergone Whipple procedures for pancreatic cancer
• Fortunately, as recognition of this condition has grown, diagnostic criteria have been created for AIP, allowing diagnosis to be made on the basis of radiologic findings and serology and confirmed by needle biopsy via ERCP, thereby sparing extensive surgical procedures in many cases

### Liver and bile ducts
• IgG4-related sclerosing cholangitis is the most common presentation of the disease in the liver
• It resembles primary sclerosing cholangitis significantly except for the response to treatment
• These patients can be treated successfully with glucocorticoids and thereby avoid rapid progression to cirrhosis with appropriate diagnosis

- Inflammatory pseudotumors of the liver, IgG4-related hepatitis, and acalculous lymphoplasmacytic cholecystitis are other IgG4-RD manifestations in the liver

## Kidney
- The clinical manifestations of IgG4-RD in the kidney consist of hematuria, proteinuria, and decreased kidney function
- Various accompanying radiologic findings include diffuse renal enlargement, focal renal masses, and thickening of the renal pelvis
- Kidney lesions are mostly found in association with other organ involvement
- IgG4-related tubulointerstitial nephritis (TIN) is the most common histologic pattern of kidney involvement
- Cases of membranous glomerulonephritis have been described in this population but whether it is secondary to immune complex deposition or due to the disease's inflammatory process is unclear

## Retroperitoneum
- More than half of the idiopathic retroperitoneal fibrosis cases have shown typical histologic findings for diagnosis of IgG4-RD in several studies
- Histologic evaluation for IgG4-RD is usually challenging in these cases because of the advanced stages of fibrosis when these lesions are biopsied
- Periaortitis and retroperitoneal fibrosis are sometimes an extension of primary aortic involvement in patients with IgG4-RD

## Lymph nodes
- Lymphadenopathy is a common finding in patients with IgG4-RD and is mostly reported in association with other organ involvement
- Generalized lymphadenopathy as a sole presentation of IgG4-RD is possible but can be a challenging diagnosis
- Lymph node histology in IgG4-RD is variable and usually does not include the storiform fibrosis
- Lack of typical histology features makes it difficult to differentiate IgG4-related lymphadenopathy from other conditions associated with elevated IgG4
    - Major conditions that need to be excluded are multicentric Castleman's disease, malignancies including lymphoma, infections, and sarcoidosis

• Making the diagnosis of IgG4-RD purely on the basis of lymph node pathology is not recommended
• Many of these patients develop other organ involvement over time, which confirms the diagnosis

## Diagnostic studies

• The diagnosis of IgG4-RD should be suspected in patients with one of the characteristic patterns of organ or tissue involvement
• Confirmation of the diagnosis is strongly suggested by biopsy and thorough evaluation of histology and immunochemistry
• The diagnosis should not be made entirely based on the number of IgG4+ plasma cells in the tissue nor on the basis of elevated serum IgG4 concentration, in the absence of compatible clinical findings

### Value of serum IgG4 in the diagnosis of IgG4-RD
• The frequency of serum IgG4 elevation in IgG4-RD varies significantly among the reported studies from 44–100%, which calls into question the value of serum IgG4 alone in the diagnosis of the disease
   ○ Some variability of this frequency maybe related to the course, activity, and treatment status of the condition at the time of sera measurement
   ○ The level of serum IgG4 elevation usually correlates with disease activity and the number of involved organs and declines after appropriate treatment with glucocorticoids
   ○ Technical issues with the IgG4 assay can also falsify the value of reported IgG4 level
• Although its elevation can be helpful for the diagnosis in the setting of characteristic organ involvement and pathology, the presence of normal serum IgG4 does not exclude the diagnosis

## Treatment

• Glucocorticoid therapy is the cornerstone of initial therapy in IgG4-RD
   ○ The response to treatment is often swift and dramatic, typically with symptomatic improvement, remarkable reduction in the size of the tumor or organ enlargement, and decline in serum IgG4 level
   ○ This response is expected if the therapy is initiated at a time before the fibroinflammatory process has become densely sclerotic
   ○ Studies have shown most patients with IgG4-RD have frequent disease relapses after tapering the glucocorticoid

• Different glucocorticoid-sparing medications have been used to treat IgG4-RD, however the exact effect of them has not been fully evaluated to establish a definitive role in IgG4-RD

• B cell depletion therapy with rituximab is regarded as an effective treatment in many patients with disease refractory to glucocorticoids and other medications

## Prognosis

• The long-term prognosis and natural history of the condition are not well defined and require dedicated long-term studies

• Patients who have localized disease confined to one organ may improve spontaneously without treatment, but many relapse in time

• Sustained remission after treatment is common; however relapses occur after discontinuation of therapy mostly in patients with multi-organ involvement and elevated serum IgG4

• Additional organs may get involved over time, despite effective treatment of initial organ involvement

• Several case reports suggest an increased risk of non-Hodgkin lymphoma among IgG4-RD patients

  ○ Additional studies are required to determine the true risk of malignancy in this population

## Further reading

Cheuk, W., Chan, J.K. (2010) IgG4-related sclerosing disease: a critical appraisal of an evolving clinicopathologic entity. *Advances in Anatomic Pathology* 17: 303–332.

Deshpande, V., Zen, Y., Ferry, J.A., et al. (2012) Consensus statement on the pathology of IgG4-related disease. *Modern Pathology* 25: 1181–1192.

Kamisawa, T., Funata, N., Hayashi, Y., et al. (2003) A new clinicopathological entity of IgG4-related autoimmune disease. *Journal of Gastroenterology* 38: 982–984.

Kamisawa, T., Okamoto, A. (2006) Autoimmune pancreatitis: proposal of IgG4-related sclerosing disease. *Journal of Gastroenterology* 41: 613–625.

Khosroshahi, A., Carruthers, M.N., Deshpande, V., et al. (2012) Rituximab for the treatment of IgG4-related disease: lessons from 10 consecutive patients. *Medicine (Baltimore)* 91: 57–66.

Khosroshahi, A., Stone, J.H. (2011) A clinical overview of IgG4-related systemic disease. *Current Opinion in Rheumatology* 23: 57–66.

Stone, J.H., Zen, Y., Deshpande, V. (2012) IgG4-related disease. *New England Journal of Medicine* 366: 539–551.

Zen, Y., Nakanuma, Y. (2010) IgG4-related disease: a cross-sectional study of 114 cases. *American Journal of Surgical Pathology* 34: 1812–1819.

## CHAPTER 6

# Myopathies

### Aliza Lipson

Emory University School of Medicine, Atlanta, GA, USA

### Introduction

Myopathies occur in both adults and children, and may be due to numerous underlying etiologies. Many of the myopathies have similar features, but appropriate classification is critical for proper management. This chapter will focus primarily on the idiopathic inflammatory myopathies and overlap syndromes, and will briefly discuss toxic myopathies.

### Common causes of myopathy

- Idiopathic inflammatory myopathies (autoimmune-mediated [AIM]): polymyositis (PM), dermatomyositis (DM), inclusion body myositis (IBM), immune-mediated necrotizing myopathy (IMNM)
- Overlap syndromes: connective tissue diseases
- Other rheumatic disease associations: sarcoidosis, IgG4
- Toxic myopathies: statin, colchicine/colcrys, alcohol, cocaine
- Endocrine: thyroid, diabetes
- Neurologic: neuropathies, dystrophies
- Mitochondrial myopathies
- Metabolic myopathies
- Cancer-associated: paraneoplastic, graft-versus-host disease (GVHD)
- Infectious: viral, human immunodeficiency virus (HIV)
- Other: eosinophilic, focal/nodular, macrophagic, granulmatous, orbital/ocular

*Rheumatology Board Review*, First Edition. Edited by Karen Law and Aliza Lipson.
© 2014 John Wiley & Sons, Inc. Published 2014 by John Wiley & Sons, Inc.

## Idiopathic inflammatory myopathies/ autoimmune-mediated (AIM)

### Epidemiology
- The AIM are the most common myopathies, but are still rare
- Annual incidence: adults: 5–10/million, children: 1–5/million
- Prevalence: 50–100 cases/million

| Keep in mind |
| --- |
| Only 60% of patients with AIM express myositis-specific autoantibodies. |

### Types of autoimmune-mediated myopathies
- **Polymyositis (PM)**
  - Pathogenesis: cytotoxic CD8+ T cells
  - Clinical presentation: weeks to months of progressive proximal muscle weakness
  - Unique features: interstitial lung disease (ILD), cardiac disease
  - Treatment response: good
- **Dermatomyositis (DM)**
  - Pathogenesis: C5b-9 MAC (membrane attack complex), CD4+ T cell perivascular inflammation
  - Clinical presentation: weeks to months of proximal muscle weakness
  - Unique features: dermatologic manifestations (see physical examination in AIM section)
  - Treatment response: good
- **Inclusion body myositis (IBM)**
  - Pathogenesis: neurodegenerative
  - Clinical presentation: years of progressive muscle weakness
  - Unique features: atrophy, asymmetric, distal weakness in addition to proximal weakness
  - Treatment response: poor, significant disability
- **Immune-mediated necrotizing myopathy (IMNM)**
  - Pathogenesis: myofiber necrosis, degeneration/regeneration, **few if any inflammatory cells**
  - Clinical presentation: not well described
  - Unique features: can be drug induced/paraneoplastic
  - Treatment response: can respond to immunosuppression

Toxic, endocrine, paraneoplastic, and muscular dystrophies can mimic inflammatory myopathies, so the **clinical picture, histopathology,** and **myositis-specific autoantibodies** must each be weighed to differentiate these syndromes.

- **Myositis associated with connective tissue disease (CTD)**
  - ○ Pathogenesis: probably a combination of mechanisms
  - ○ Clinical presentation: generally proximal muscle weakness, plus features of CTD
  - ○ Typically associated with:
    - ▪ Scleroderma (16–93%)
    - ▪ Lupus
    - ▪ Mixed connective tissue disease (MCTD)
    - ▪ Sjögrens
    - ▪ Rheumatoid arthritis
  - ○ Symptoms may be mild to severe
- **Juvenile polymositis/dermatomyositis**
  - ○ Pathogenesis: similar to adult
  - ○ Clinical presentation: similar to adult presentation, however DM is more common
  - ○ Unique features: painful subcutaneous calcifications can occur, and tend to be more common in pediatric populations
- **Amyopathic dermatomyositis**
  - ○ Pathogenesis: same as DM
  - ○ Clinical presentation:
    - ▪ Skin manifestations **without** muscle disease or elevated muscle enzymes
    - ▪ ILD
    - ▪ May be associated with pneumothoraces or pneumomediastinum

### Classification criteria
The original criteria were defined by Bohan and Peter in 1975.
- These were devised prior to the discovery of myositis-specific antibodies and the recognition of IBM as a separate disease entity
- Patients were assessed by the following criteria:
  - ○ Symmetric, proximal muscle weakness
  - ○ Rash typical of DM
  - ○ Elevated muscle enzymes

○ Myopathic changes on electromyography (EMG)

○ Characteristic muscle biopsy without signs of other myopathies

• Based on the pattern of the above, patients were divided into either probable or definite inflammatory myopathy

## International Myositis Assessment and Clinical Studies Group (IMACS)

• Due to the complex nature of myopathies, the IMACS is making efforts to characterize the AIM (Table 6.1) by using a combination of clinical, serologic, histopathological markers, with the production of definite criteria underway

---

**Keep in mind**

Classification of the idiopathic inflammatory myopathies continues to evolve.

---

## Physical examination in AIM

• **Neurologic**

○ Weakness in proximal muscle groups of upper and lower extremities, neck flexors

○ Muscle pain is not a primary feature

○ Distal weakness is characteristic of IBM

○ Muscle atrophy is characteristic of IBM or late PM/DM

○ Note: a patient presenting with weakness over years, asymmetric/distal/facial weakness and scapular winging should prompt evaluation for dystrophy, not myopathy, as a cause of their weakness

• **Musculoskeletal**

○ Synovitis can be present in overlap syndromes

• **Dermatologic** (primarily seen in DM)

○ Heliotrope rash: violaceous papules around eyes

○ Gottron papules: erythematous papules, plaques over MCPs, PIPs, DIPs

○ Poikiloderma/photosensitive erythematous rash characterized by location:

**Table 6.1** Summary of classification considerations for AIM, incorporating clinical, serologic and histopathologic components.

| | Polymyositis | Dermatomyositis | Inclusion body myositis | Immune-mediated necrotizing myopathy |
|---|---|---|---|---|
| **Pathogenesis** | Autoimmune, inflammatory | Autoimmune, inflammatory | Myodegenerative >> inflammatory | Necrosis >> inflammatory |
| **Clinical presentation** | Subacute symmetric **proximal** muscle weakness (weeks to months) Painless, although myalgias common | Subacute symmetric **proximal** muscle weakness (weeks to months) Painless, although myalgias common | Slowly progressive **proximal and distal** muscle weakness; **muscle atrophy** | Weeks to months of myalgias, weakness |
| **Treatment response and prognosis** | Good 5 yr survival 75–95% | Good 5 yr adult survival 75–90% 5 yr pediatric survival >95% | Poor 5 year survival 100%, but with disability | Poor |
| **Other organ involvement** | Yes 5–46% (ILD, cardiac) | Yes 5–46% (ILD, cardiac) | No | Yes, if paraneoplastic |
| **Myositis-specific autoantibodies** | Yes | Yes | No | Yes |
| **Age of onset** | Age 30–50 years | Age 7 years; age 30–50 years | Older men | Varies |
| **Muscle biopsy** | Cytotoxic CD8+ T cells surrounding and invading non-necrotic myofibers | Atrophic, degenerating and regenerating fibers, CD4+ T cells in a perivascular pattern | Rimmed vacuoles | Necrotic muscle infiltrated by macrophages |

Although the prevalence of ILD in some of these groups can range from 5–46%, ILD may be asymptomatic

- Shawl sign: upper back
- V sign: sun-exposed areas of upper chest
- Holster sign: lateral thighs

o Nail bed changes: periungual telangiectasias, cuticular hypertrophy

o Mechanics' hands: rough, cracked skin over fingertips and lateral aspect of fingers, most commonly seen in antisynthetase syndrome

o Skin changes are typically very photosensitive

o Painful subcutaneous calcifications can also occur, seen primarily in juvenile DM and CTD overlap syndromes

o If dermatologic signs are seen without evidence of associated muscle disease, these patients are categorized as amyopathic dermatomyositis

## Laboratory findings in AIM

- Muscle enzymes
  o Creatine kinase (CK): most sensitive and specific
  o Aldolase: can be elevated in isolation
  o Lactate dehydrogenase (LDH)
- Aspartate transaminase (AST)
- Alanine transaminase (ALT)
- **Normal thyroid studies are needed to exclude thyroid disease as a cause of myopathy**

### Keep in mind

Unnecessary liver biopsies are sometimes done when elevations in liver enzymes are seen due to **inflammatory muscle disease**, not liver disease. In these situations, **gamma-glutamyl transpeptidase** (GGT) can be helpful to differentiate between muscle or intrinsic liver disease, as GGT is present in liver but not muscle.

- **Autoantibodies**
  o DM and PM generally are seronegative (negative ANA, RF), but low titer positivity can be seen
  o **Myositis-associated autoantibodies** (Table 6.2)
    - These autoantibodies are primarily directed against nucleolar targets
    - Typically seen in **myositis-associated CTD**/overlap syndromes
  o **Myositis-specific autoantibodies** (Table 6.3)

- Target: nuclear or cytoplasmic components involved in gene transcription, protein translocation, and antiviral response
- Seen almost exclusively in **immune-mediated myopathies** (60–80% of patients with AIM have associated autoantibodies)
- ○ **Additional myositis-associated autoantibodies** (Table 6.4)
    - Many other autoantibodies have been reported with varying prevalence and disease associations
    - Given their relatively low prevalence and varying availability, routine evaluation with these antibodies in all patients with myopathy may be costly and low-yield
    - In patients in whom a diagnosis is unclear after extensive workup, evaluating for the presence of these antibodies may have a role

**Table 6.2** Myositis-associated autoantibodies.

| Autoantibody | Antigen | Location | Clinically available | CTD |
|---|---|---|---|---|
| Anti-Ro Anti-La | 60KD/52KD 48KD | Nucleus | Yes | Sjögren's |
| Anti-U1-RNP | U1 RNA | Nucleus | Yes | MCTD |
| Anti-PM-Scl | PM-Scl 75 and PM-Scl 100 | Nucleus | | Scleroderma |
| Anti-Ku | 60-66KD,80-86KD | Nucleus and Cytoplasm | | Overlap |

**Table 6.3** Myositis-specific autoantibodies.

| Antisynthetase autoantibodies | Antigen | Location | Inflammatory myopathy association | Clinically available | PM/DM |
|---|---|---|---|---|---|
| Anti-Jo-1 | Histidyl-tRNA-synthetase | Cytoplasm | Antisynthetase syndrome | Yes | 25–30% |
| Anti-PL12, PL7, EJ, OJ, Zo | Various aminoacyl-tRNA-synthetases | Cytoplasm | Antisynthetase syndrome | Less | 1–5% |

Table 6.4 Additional myositis-associated autoantibodies.

| Nonsynthetase autoantibodies | Antigen | Target location | Inflammatory myopathy association |
| --- | --- | --- | --- |
| Anti-SRP | RNP complex | Cytoplasm | IMNM<br>Rapidly progressive, systemic features<br>May be refractory<br>Rare in pediatrics |
| Anti-Mi-2 | DNA helicase<br>Transcriptional repressor | Nucleus | DM only (20%)<br>More severe cutaneous<br>Better response to therapy<br>Decrease malignancy risk<br>Adults and pediatrics |
| Anti-HMGCR | HMGCoa reductase | | Statin-induced IMNM |
| Anti-MDA5 | | | Amyopathic DM, progressive ILD |
| Anti-p155/140 | Transcriptional intermediary factor | Nucleus | Increased malignancy risk adults<br>Severe cutaneous disease |
| Anti-MJ | | | JDM only<br>Increased risk of calcinosis |
| Anti-p140 | Nuclear transcription protein | Nucleus | JDM with calcinosis |
| Anti-SAE | | | Adult DM, can be cancer associated |
| Anti-CADM-140 | MDA5 gene (melanoma differentiation-associated gene 5)<br>Innate response to viral infection | Cytoplasm | Cancer associated<br>Cutaneous > muscle involvement<br>Rapidly progressive<br>ILD |

**Antisynthetase syndrome** is a subset of AIM with several classic features. Identification of this syndrome has important prognostic implications, as these patients typically have rapidly progressive disease manifestations.
- Autoimmune myopathy
- Interstitial lung disease
- Non-erosive arthritis
- Fever
- Mechanics' hands: hyperkeratotic lesions lateral and palmar aspects of fingers
- Antisynthetase autoantibodies (i.e. Anti Jo-1)

- **Genetic markers**
  - A genetic contribution is recognized, but extent is not well known due to small sample size
  - Multi-genic, multi-mechanistic pathways have been described
  - HLA-B8/DR3/DR52/DQ2 are associated with IBM
- **Electromyography and nerve conduction study (EMG/NCS)**
  - Results may vary and may be operator-dependent unless standardized techniques are used
  - Must consider timing during a patient's workup and treatment; attempt to have EMG performed prior to or soon after starting corticosteroids to ensure the most accurate results
  - Typical findings in AIM:
    - Increased **insertional activity, fibrillations**, and **sharp positive waves**
    - **Polyphasic motor-unit potentials** of low amplitude and short duration
    - Spontaneous, bizarre, **high-frequency discharges**
  - Complete triad is seen in ~40% of patients
  - 10% of patients with AIM may have a normal EMG
- **Muscle biopsy**

*"[Muscle biopsies show] degenerating and/or necrotic myofibers, regenerating muscle fibers, atrophic muscle cells and evidence of inflammatory infiltrate."*
*Peter and Bohan, 1975*

  - The original Peter and Bohan histopathololologic description of inflammatory myopathies is no longer specific enough to be used clinically

- The findings originally described may be seen in AIM, IBM or even some dystrophies.
  - Muscle biopsies are categorized by three major components:
    - Histological/histochemical
    - Myopathic vs. neuropathic patterns of disease
    - Presence of unique features that are clues to underlying patho-physiology and diagnosis
  - **Myopathic pattern**
    - Rounding and variation of myofiber size
    - Internal nuclei, fiber atrophy, denenerating and regenerating myofibers
    - Fatty replacement
  - **Neuropathic pattern**
    - Evidence of denervation and re-innervation
    - Small, atrophic, angular fibers and target fibers
    - Re-innveration results in fiber type grouping
  - **Unique features**
    - **Dermatomyositis**
      - → Perifascicular atrophy, degenerating/regenerating myofibers
      - → These findings are caused by infiltration of C5b-9 MAC leading to capillary dropout causing ischemia of myofibers
      - → Perivascular inflammation comprised of B cells, CD4+ T cells, and plasmacytoid dendritic cells
    - **Polymyositis**
      - → Cytotoxic CD8+ T cells and macrophages are present, surround-ing and invading non-necrotic myofibers
    - **Inclusion body myositis**: presence of rimmed vacuoles
    - **Immune-mediated necrotizing myopathy**: myofiber necrosis, degeneration, and regeneration, with scant or no inflammatory cells
  - Special considerations with muscle biopsies:
    - Muscle necrosis can be seen in IMNM, toxic, endocrine, and para-neoplastic myopathies, as well as dystrophies; myositis-specific autoantibodies can be helpful in this regard
    - Due to the site-specific/patchy nature of many of the myopathies, blind muscle biopsies have a >12% false-negative rate
    - Obtain muscle biopsies and EMG/NCS prior to the use of gluco-corticoids, if possible, as steroids can affect the results of these tests
- **Skin biopsy**
  - **Dermatomyositis**
    - Inflammatory cells at dermo-epidermal junction, "interface dermatitis"

- Inflammatory cells around small blood vessels in dermis
- Mucin deposition
- Lupus skin biopsy may have a similar appearance

- **Magnetic resonance imaging (MRI)** findings in myopathy
  - Increased signal intensity within muscle tissue
  - May see muscle necrosis, degeneration, and/or inflammation
  - May see fatty replacement, an indicator of chronic muscle damage (poor response to therapy)
  - Findings may help guide site selection for muscle biopsy
  - MRI offers a less invasive assessment tool in pediatric populations
  - MRI can help assess clinical response, though criteria for this have yet to be fully established

## Treatment

- **Pharmacologic**
  - **Glucocorticoids**: PO/IV 1 mg/kg, tapering after 4 weeks
    - Be aware with chronic steroid use that **steroid myopathy** may also cause weakness (typically without muscle enzyme elevations)
  - **Non-glucocorticoid**
    - Methotrexate
    - Azathioprine
    - IVIG – proven efficacy in DM populations
    - Mycophenolate mofetil
    - Cyclosporine
    - Tacrolimus
    - Cyclophosphamide
    - Rituximab
    - Anti-TNFs
    - Selection of second-line treatment must be tailored to specific patient characteristics and comorbidities
    - Multiple steroid-sparing agents have been used with moderate success, but sometimes multiple regimens must be tried before finding the treatment that affords optimal response in an individual patient
    - Stem cell transplant has been studied, but has not yet shown compelling evidence of efficacy

- **Non-pharmacologic**
  - Physical therapy is critical to rebuild muscle mass, especially as muscle enzymes return to normal in response to treatment
  - Skin protective measures and avoidance of UV light in dermatomyositis

# Other considerations in myopathies

## Cancer-associated myositis
- Due to expression of similar autoantigens in both cancer tissue and muscle tissue
- Peak incidence within 2 years preceding or following myopathy diagnosis
- DM>>PM>>IBM in cancer-associated myositis
- Anti-155/140 Ab is often present
- Most common malignancies include adenocarcinoma of the cervix, lung, ovary, pancreas, bladder, and stomach, though many other cancers have been reported
- **Recommendations for malignancy screening**
  - Age-appropriate cancer screening (if delinquent) should be pursued once an inflammatory myopathy is diagnosed
  - Chest, abdomen, and pelvis imaging, endoscopy/colonoscopy, brain imaging, bone marrow biopsy, etc. are not routinely recommended but may be indicated in symptomatic patients or patients with refractory myopathy

## Toxic and drug-induced myopathies
- **Statin-induced**
  - Statins cause a spectrum of muscle manifestations ranging from myalgias → myositis → necrotizing myopathy
  - Target: autoAb 3-hydroxy-3-methylglutaryl-coenzyme A reductase
  - Some patients may continue to manifest symptoms of muscle pain and weakness up to 6–8 months after the statin is withheld
- **Colchicine**
  - Neuromyopathy can develop after an acutely large dose or chronic low dose
  - Reversible, with myopathy recovery faster than neuropathy
  - Chronic kidney disease (CKD) is a risk factor for colchicine toxicity
- **Steroid myopathy**
  - Lab evaluation shows normal CK and other muscle enzymes
  - EMG is usually normal, but may reveal low-amplitude motor unit potentials
  - Non-specific atrophy of type IIb muscle fibers is seen on muscle biopsy
  - Reversible with reduction/discontinuation of steroids

- **Alcohol**
  - Acute alcoholic myopathy induces asymptomatic CK elevaton and rhabdomyolysis, propagated by hypophosphatemia and hypokalemia
  - Chronic alcoholic myopathy presents with weeks to months of proximal muscle weakness, with normal to mild elevation of CK
- **Cocaine**
  - Asymptomatic CK elevation can lead to rhabdomyolysis
- **Nucleoside reverse transcriptase inhibitors**
  - Myopathy typically presents with proximal muscle weakness and myalgias
  - Causes a specific type of mitochondrial myopathy
  - Patients may have elevated CK, and occasionally abnormal EMG
  - Can be reversible when diagnosed and treated early

## Myopathy associated with hypothyroidism

- Myalgia, not weakness, is the primary complaint
- Elevated CK (<10× normal) may lead to rhabdomyolysis in rare cases
- Additional features include proximal myopathy, muscle hypertrophy, and myoedema (sustained muscle contracture due to delayed relaxation phase)

## Further reading

Bohan, A., Peter, J.B. (1975) Polymyositis and dermatomyositis (first of two parts). *New England Journal of Medicine* 292: 344.

Bohan, A., Peter, J.B. (1975) Polymyositis and dermatomyositis (second of two parts). *New England Journal of Medicine* 292: 403.

Isenberg, D.A., Allen, E., Farewell, V., et al.; for the International Myositis and Clinical Studies Group (IMACS) (2003) International consensus outcome measures for patients with idiopathic inflammatory myopathies: development and initial validation of myositis activity and damage indices in patients with adult onset disease. *Rheumatology (Oxford)* 42: 1–7.

IMACS official consensus statement is in process. Relevant sources for further reading may be found at: http://rwd.niehs.nih.gov/rwd/research/resources/collab/imacs/imacspubs/index.cfm

# CHAPTER 7

# Selected topics in pediatric rheumatology

**Sampath Prahalad, Sheila Angeles-Han, Kelly A. Rouster-Stevens, Larry Vogler**

Emory University School of Medicine, Children's Healthcare of Atlanta, Atlanta, GA, USA

## Introduction

Rheumatic diseases in pediatric populations require special considerations. While some features are similar in adult populations, others such as the juvenile idiopathic arthritides have different classification criteria and approaches to diagnosis. Manifestations in young patients have unique features as well as pediatric-specific treatment considerations. This chapter will review considerations in juvenile idiopathic arthritis, pediatric systemic lupus erythematosus, juvenile dermatomyositis, and the childhood vasculitides.

## Juvenile idiopathic arthritis (JIA)

- Juvenile idiopathic arthritis refers to a collection of chronic arthropathies in children
- Several clinically and genetically distinct subtypes are recognized
- While the pathophysiology of JIA is complex, both genetic and environmental factors are believed to play a role in the susceptibility to JIA
  - JIA is a heterogeneous collection of chronic arthritis in children
  - All subtypes of JIA have in common arthritis in one or more joints for at least 6 weeks in a child under the age of 16 years
  - Different subtypes of JIA have different clinical features, genetic associations, comorbidities, and outcomes

*Rheumatology Board Review*, First Edition. Edited by Karen Law and Aliza Lipson.
© 2014 John Wiley & Sons, Inc. Published 2014 by John Wiley & Sons, Inc.

## Epidemiology
- JIA is the most common childhood rheumatic disease encountered in pediatric rheumatology clinics
- The incidence of JIA is 1 in 10,000 children; prevalence is approximately 1 in 1000 children under 16 years
- Most subtypes of JIA are more common in girls than in boys

## Classification and diagnosis
- JIA is a heterogeneous disease with several subtypes
- Historically the terms juvenile rheumatoid arthritis (JRA) and juvenile chronic arthritis (JCA) have been used to describe and classify chronic arthritis in childhood
  - Each of these classifications included different subtypes, which resulted in difficulties in comparing studies from Europe and the US
  - Consequently the International League of Associations for Rheumatology (ILAR) criteria were developed which are comprehensive and more uniform
- The American College of Rheumatology Criteria defined juvenile rheumatoid arthritis (JRA) as arthritis in one or more joints for at least 6 weeks in a child under 16 years
  - Pauciarticular JRA is arthritis in four or fewer joints in the first 6 months of disease
  - Polyarticular JRA is arthritis in five or more joints in the first 6 months of disease
  - Systemic JRA is daily (quotidian) fever spiking to more than 39 °C for at least 2 weeks in association with arthritis in one or more joints
- The European League Against Rheumatism (EULAR) criteria recognized juvenile chronic arthritis (JCA) as arthritis in one or more joints for at least 3 months in a child under 16 years
  - Systemic JCA is arthritis with characteristic fever
  - Polyarticular JCA is arthritis in more than four joints with negative rheumatoid factor
  - Juvenile rheumatoid arthritis is arthritis in more than four joints with positive rheumatoid factor
  - Pauciarticular JCA is arthritis in fewer than five joints
  - Juvenile ankylosing spondylitis is the presence of features of ankylosing spondylitis in a child younger than 16 years
  - Juvenile psoriatic arthritis is the presence or psoriatic arthritis in a child younger than 16 years

- The International League of Associations for Rheumatology (ILAR) criteria form the most current classification system for JIA
  - The ILAR criteria define JIA as arthritis in one or more joints for at least 6 weeks in a child under 16 years
  - The ILAR criteria specified **exclusion criteria** to define homogeneous, mutually exclusive subtypes of JIA as follows:
    (a) Psoriasis or a history of psoriasis in the patient or first-degree relative
    (b) Arthritis in an HLA-B27 positive male after the 6th birthday
    (c) Ankylosing spondylitis, enthesitis-related arthritis, sacroiliitis with inflammatory bowel disease, Reiter's syndrome or acute anterior uveitis, or a history of one of these disorders in a first-degree relative
    (d) The presence of IgM rheumatoid factor on at least two occasions at least 3 months apart
    (e) The presence of systemic JIA
  - The ILAR criteria classify JIA into seven subtypes:
    - In **systemic JIA** there is arthritis in one or more joints with fever of at least 2 weeks' duration accompanied by one of the following: evanescent rash, serositis, lymphadenopathy or hepatosplenomegaly
      → Exclusions: a, b, c, d
      → Systemic JIA affects boys and girls equally
      → Systemic JIA makes up 4–17% of all JIA
    - **Oligoarticular JIA** affects one to four joints during the first 6 months of disease
      → Exclusions: a, b, c, d, e
      → Two subcategories are recognized
        - Persistent oligoarthritis affects up to four joints throughout the course of the disease
        - Extended oligoarthritis affects more than four joints after the first 6 months of disease
      → Oligoarticular JIA affects girls more often than boys
      → It is the most common subtype of JIA, 27–56% of all JIA
      → Onset is typically in early childhood, peak 2–4 years
    - **Polyarthritis (rheumatoid factor (RF)-negative)** presents with arthritis affecting five or more joints during the first 6 months of disease
      → Exclusions: a, b, c, d, e
      → A test for RF is negative
      → RF-negative polyarticular JIA affects girls more often than boys

→ It is the second most common subtype of JIA, 11–28% of all JIA
→ Onset is biphasic, early peak at 2–4 and later peak at 6–12 years
→ Uveitis can be seen with this subtype as well

- **Polyarthritis (RF positive)** affects five or more joints during the first 6 months of disease
  → Exclusions: a, c, d, e
  → This is typically seen in older children and teens
  → It is much more common among females
  → Two or more tests for RF at least 3 months apart during the first 6 months of disease are positive
  → Most children are also positive for anti-CCP antibodies
  → This subtype makes up ~2–7% of all JIA
  → It can be associated with rheumatoid nodules
  → This subtype has the potential for aggressive disease and poor outcome
  → Uveitis is rare with this subtype

- **Psoriatic arthritis** is arthritis **and** psoriasis, or arthritis and at least two of the following:
  - Dactylitis
  - Nail pitting
  - Onycholysis
  - Family history of psoriasis (in a first-degree relative)
  → Exclusions: b, c, d, e
  → This subtype makes up 2–11% of all JIA

- **Enthesitis-related arthritis** (ERA) is diagnosed if there is arthritis **and/or** enthesitis with at least two of the following:
  - Presence of or history of sacroiliac joint tenderness with or without inflammatory lumbosacral pain
  - Presence of HLA-B27 antigen
  - Onset of arthritis in a male over 6 years of age
  - Acute (symptomatic) anterior uveitis
  - History of ankylosing spondylitis, enthesitis-related arthritis, sacroiliitis with inflammatory bowel disease, Reiter's syndrome, or acute anterior uveitis in a first-degree relative
  → Exclusions: a, d, e
  → This subtype affects boys much more than girls
  → This subtype is associated with acute, painful uveitis
  → ERA makes up 3–11% of all JIA, and typically presents in late childhood or adolescence

■ **Undifferentiated arthritis** is arthritis that does not fulfill criteria in any of the above categories or that fulfills criteria for two or more of the above categories
    → About 11–21% of children in various series have been reported to have undifferentiated JIA

## Comorbid conditions

- **Chronic anterior uveitis**
  - Chronic anterior uveitis is seen in about 10–20% of children with JIA
  - Onset is insidious and often asymptomatic
  - Risk of chronic anterior uveitis is higher in those children with positive ANA, and younger age of onset, and in the first 4 years of disease
  - Children with JIA are advised to undergo regular slit lamp examinations by an ophthalmologist to detect and treat uveitis promptly
  - Untreated uveitis can lead to irregular pupils, glaucoma, cataracts, and vision loss
  - The risk of chronic anterior uveitis is highest among those children with oligoarticular and JIA, affecting up to 30% of patients
  - Children with RF-negative polyarthritis and psoriatic arthritis are also at risk of chronic anterior uveitis, especially if they are ANA positive
  - Children with systemic JIA seldom develop uveitis
  - Treatment includes topical steroids initially, and, for refractory disease, systemic medications are used

- **Acute uveitis**
  - In contrast to children with chronic anterior uveitis, children with acute uveitis tend to be symptomatic
  - It presents typically with eye pain, photophobia, redness
  - Unless promptly seen by an ophthalmologist, symptoms are often attributed to foreign body, infection or allergy
  - It is usually unilateral and often recurrent
  - Typically uveitis resolves without leaving sequelae
  - Visual prognosis is typically excellent
  - In a large series, 7.8% of children with ERA had acute uveitis

- **Macrophage activation syndrome (MAS)/hemophagocytic lymphohistiocytosis (HLH)**
  - This is a rare and potentially lethal condition
  - Up to 7% of children with systemic JIA may develop MAS/HLH over the course of their illness

○ MAS often follows an infection, particularly by members of the herpesvirus family such as Epstein Barr virus

○ Clinically characterized by rapid development of an unremitting fever, hepatosplenomegaly, lymphadenopathy, hepatic dysfunction, encephalopathy, purpura, bruising, and mucosal bleeding

○ More severely affected children can develop multi-organ failure

○ Laboratory features include the following

- Leukopenia
- Thrombocytopenia
- Anemia
- A sudden and paradoxical drop in erythrocyte sedimentation rate (ESR), with an elevated C-reactive protein (CRP)
- Abnormal prothrombin time (PT), partial thromboplastin time (PTT)
- Elevated fibrin degradation products and fall in fibrinogen
- Elevations of aspartate aminotransferase (AST) and alanine aminotransferase (ALT)
- Significant elevation of ferritin and soluble IL2 receptor levels

○ Demonstration of prominent phagocytosis of other hematopoietic cells by macrophages in the bone marrow, lymph nodes, liver, or spleen is diagnostic

○ Treatment includes high-dose intravenous steroids and cyclosporine

○ Cases refractory to treatment or severe presentations should prompt treatment according to the HLH protocol with corticosteroids, cyclosporine, and etoposide

- **Long-term sequelae**: children who have a delayed diagnosis or have poorly controlled JIA are at risk for some long-term sequelae

  ○ Leg length disturbances
  - Typically seen in children with asymmetric oligoarticular JIA with unilateral knee involvement
  - The affected limb tends to be longer due to hyperemia
  - This requires shoe-lift or orthotics to correct gait abnormalities

  ○ Micrognathia
  - Children with JIA who have disease of the temporomandibular joints are at risk for micrognathia

  ○ Cervical spine fusion
  - Children with involvement of cervical spine joints can develop fusion of the posterior elements of the cervical spine
  - This results in decreased range of motion of the neck, and a potential for cervical spine subluxation with hyperextension of the neck such as during anesthesia

○ Erosions
  ▪ Poorly controlled or active arthritis can result in cartilage loss, which presents as joint space narrowing on radiographs, and later bony erosions
  ▪ This can cause pain and disability
○ Growth retardation
  ▪ Although rare, long standing active arthritis, in particular systemic JIA, can result in growth delays and retardation

## Laboratory tests in JIA

- **Anti-nuclear antibodies (ANA)**
  ○ ANA may be positive in ~60% of children with JIA
  ○ ANA tend to be higher among children with oligoarticular JIA and RF-negative polyarticular JIA
  ○ ANA are rare among children with systemic JIA or ERA
  ○ Positive ANA are associated with a higher risk for chronic anterior uveitis
  ○ Most often the ANA, when positive, are of low to moderate titer
  ○ Tests for Smith, RNP, SSA, SSB, and ds-DNA are typically negative
  ○ ANA-positive JIA patients have been reported to constitute a homogeneous population despite differences in ILAR-recognized subtypes
- **Rheumatoid factor (RF)**
  ○ Children with RF-positive polyarticular JIA by definition have positive tests for IgM-RF
  ○ The ILAR criteria require the presence of two positive tests for RF in the first 6 months, at least 3 months apart
  ○ Positive RF is associated with potential for poor outcome
  ○ False-positive IgM-RF can be seen with infections, but these typically resolve; hence the requirement for two positive RF tests
- **Anti-citrullinated peptide antibodies (ACPA)**
  ○ Antibodies to citrullinated peptide antibodies are highly specific for adult-seropositive RA
  ○ The most widely available commercial test assays for antibodies to cyclic citrullinated peptides (CCP)
  ○ Most children with RF-positive JIA are also positive for anti-CCP antibodies
  ○ Anti-CCP antibodies may appear prior to clinical manifestation of inflammatory arthritis
- **HLA-B27**
  ○ HLA-B27 is a polymorphic form of the gene encoding human leukocyte antigen class I molecule – HLA B

○ HLA-B27 is associated with ankylosing spondylitis or spondyloarthropathy

○ A positive test for HLA-B27 is observed in ~7% of white northern European population in the US

○ The frequency of HLA-B27 is lower among African and African-American individuals

○ A positive HLA-B27 is found in 80–90% of children with enthesitis-related arthritis

- **Complete blood count (CBC)**
  ○ CBC is often obtained as a baseline lab test in children with JIA
  ○ With oligoarticular JIA and many children with RF-negative polyarticular JIA, CBC is often normal
  ○ Children with systemic JIA typically present with leukocytosis, thrombocytopenia, and anemia
  ○ Children with ERA might have anemia
- **Comprehensive metabolic panel (CMP)**
  ○ CMP is also obtained as a baseline lab test in children with JIA
  ○ Children with systemic JIA may have hypoalbuminemia
  ○ Most children with JIA do not have abnormal CMP
  ○ Since there can be alterations of AST and ALT with some of the medications used to treat JIA, a baseline evaluation is recommended
  ○ **Elevated AST and ALT in systemic JIA could indicate macrophage activation syndrome**

## Treatment
- **Non-steroidal anti inflammatory drugs** (NSAIDs)
  ○ NSAIDs are often the first line of treatment of JIA
  ○ Ibuprofen is used at a dose of 30 mg/kg/day in three divided doses
  ○ Naproxen is one of the commonly used NSAIDs at doses of 15–20 mg/kg/day in two divided doses with a maximum of 500 mg BID
  ○ Meloxicam can also be used as a single daily dose at 0.25 mg/kg/day with a maximum of 15 mg daily
  ○ Other agents used are nabumetone (30 mg/kg/day in one to two doses; maximum 2000 mg/day) and indocin (1.5–3 mg/kg/day; maximum 200 mg/day)
  ○ Celecoxib is a COX-2 inhibitor that can also be used in some children intolerant to the other NSAID agents
  ○ All NSAIDs can cause gastritis, so it is recommended that they be taken with food, and if indicated be used with H2-receptor blockers or proton pump inhibitors
  ○ NSAIDs can also case **acute renal papillary necrosis**, which can present with hematuria

○ Naproxen can cause **pseudoporphyria** and increased skin fragility, especially in fair-skinned individuals

- **Steroids**
  ○ Steroids are often used as bridge agents to achieve short-term disease control
  ○ They are most useful in the setting of systemic JIA
  ○ For serositis or MAS, intravenous steroids are indicated
  ○ Low-dose steroids may also have a role in polyarticular JIA, especially with positive RF
  ○ Steroids have many side effects with prolonged usage including notably weight gain, osteoporosis, hypertension, hyperglycemia, cataracts, striae
  ○ Prednisone is often used at doses ranging from 0.5–2 mg/kg/day
  ○ For children with oligoarticular JIA, and for some children with other types of JIA, intra-articular injection of steroids is a very effective form of treatment
  ○ The most commonly employed agent is triamcinolone hexacetonide which has a long half-life
  ○ Children with uveitis/iritis typically are treated with topical steroid drops, and in some instances intra-ocular depot steroid preparations

- **Methotrexate**
  ○ Methotrexate is the preferred agent employed as a disease-modifying antirheumatic drug (DMARD)
  ○ It is indicated in polyarticular JIA, systemic JIA with predominantly articular features, extended oligoarticular JIA, and in persistent oligoarticular JIA with poor response to NSAIDs and/or intra-articular steroids
  ○ It is available as tablets for oral form or injection for parenteral use, typically administered subcutaneously
  ○ The usual starting dose of 0.5 mg/kg given once weekly, and increased as tolerated to 1 mg/kg/week; we recommend using up to a maximum of 25 mg/wk in most children
  ○ Beyond 20 mg/week, most clinicians prefer to use it subcutaneously
  ○ Adverse effects
    ▪ Most children tolerate methotrexate without problems
    ▪ In some children methotrexate can cause nausea which can occur from just before the dose up to 24–48 hours after the dose.
    ▪ Methotrexate can also cause oral mucosal ulcers (mucositis) at higher doses
      → Folic acid given daily at 1 mg can minimize oral ulcers

- Methotrexate can also cause elevations in AST and ALT, as well as leukopenia
  ○ The ACR recommends CBC, CMP prior to initiating methotrexate, 1–2 months after starting or after dose change, and every 2–3 months on stable doses
  ○ Methotrexate is potentially teratogenic and female patients taking this drug should be counseled against getting pregnant while on it
- **Leflunomide**
  ○ Leflunomide is an immunomodulatory agent that inhibits pyrimidine synthesis
  ○ It is considered for patients who do not tolerate methotrexate
  ○ Usually administered with a loading dose, followed by every day or every other day dosing depending on the weight of the child
  ○ Improvement should be notable by 6–12 weeks
  ○ CBC, WBC count, differential, platelet count, AST, ALT, and albumin should be monitored every 4–12 weeks
  ○ Leflunomide is teratogenic
    - It has a long half-life, and it has been recommended that cholestyramine be administered and drug levels be verified to be less than 0.02 mg/L on at least two occasions, 2 weeks apart in individuals wishing to conceive
- **Biological response modifiers**
  ○ TNF inhibitors
    - Tumor necrosis factor (TNF-α) is a pro-inflammatory cytokine found in elevated levels in individuals with JIA and RA as well as other inflammatory disorders
    - Biological agents that antagonize TNF-α have been shown to be effective in the treatment of JIA
    - Currently two anti-TNF agents are approved for use in JIA
      → **Etanercept** is given once or twice weekly subcutaneously at 0.8 mg/kg/week
      → **Adalimumab** is given once every other week subcutaneously at 0.4 mL (20 mg) for children <30 kg and 0.8 mL (40 mg) for children >30 kg
      → In addition, **infliximab** is also used by many clinicians, given as intravenous infusions at doses 3–10 mg/kg given every 4–8 weeks
      → Other anti-TNF agents approved for use in adults with RA are being investigated in children at this time
    - All TNF inhibitors have potential to increase susceptibility to serious infections including mycobacterial and fungal infections

- A test for tuberculosis (PPD or Quantiferon gold) is recommended prior to initiating anti-TNF therapy and annual screening for TB is recommended
- Children with serious infections are advised to hold TNF inhibitors until their primary infection has been adequately treated
- Most children tolerate anti-TNF agents well; some develop injection site or infusion reactions

○ **Tocilizumab**

- Tocilizumab is a monoclonal antibody directed against IL-6, which is a potent proinflammatory cytokine
- Tocilizumab has been approved for the treatment of systemic JIA and polyarticular JIA
- It is given as an intravenous infusion every 2 weeks for systemic JIA and every 4 weeks for polyarticular JIA
- The dose is 8 mg/kg/dose, and for children less than 30 kg, the dose is 12 mg/kg/dose
- Major adverse events include infusion reactions, cytopenias, increased liver transaminases, and hypercholesterolemia
- Tocilizumab can be given with methotrexate
- Tocilizumab is also effective in treating adult RA

○ **Anakinra**

- Anakinra is a human recombinant form of IL-1 receptor antagonist produced by recombinant technology in *Escherichia coli*
- Anakinra has shown improvement in features of JIA compared to placebo, although the improvements were not as dramatic as with TNF inhibitors
- Anakinra appears to be particularly effective in the treatment of systemic JIA especially in children with predominantly systemic features
- The commonly used dose for anakinra is 1 mg/kg increased to 2 mg/kg (maximum of 100 mg)
- Side effects include injection site reactions and increased susceptibility to infections
- Although not associated with reactivation of latent TB, documenting a negative PPD before initiating treatment is recommended
- Improvement is often seen with within 2 weeks
- Neutrophil count should be monitored at baseline, monthly for 3 months and then quarterly

○ **Abatacept**

- Abatacept is a fully human, soluble fusion protein which prevents a co-stimulatory signal necessary for T cell activation

- It binds to CD80 and CD86, thereby blocking interaction with CD28, which results in downregulation of the antigen presenting cell–T lymphocyte interaction
- It is available as an infusion which has a pediatric indication for JIA
- Recently a subcutaneous formulation of abatacept has been marketed
- Most common side effects are headaches, upper respiratory tract infections, nasopharyngitis, and nausea
- Dose: for patients less than 75 kg, the dose is 10 mg/kg IV, 75–100 kg dose is 750 mg IV, and >100 kg: 1000 mg
- It is given intravenously over 30 minutes on week 0, 2, 4, and every 4 weeks
- Abatacept is generally effective and well tolerated
- Abatacept also showed efficacy in a trial of subjects that failed previous biological therapy
- Can be administered with methotrexate

○ **Rituximab**
- Rituximab is a chimeric monoclonal mouse–human antibody targeting the CD20 receptor on mature B cells and pre B cells, but not stem cells of plasma cells
- Rituximab exerts its effects by removing B cells from circulation and is theoretically beneficial in diseases where autoantibodies may be pathogenically important
- It is indicated for adults with RA
- It is commonly used for children with RF-positive polyarticular JIA who are refractory to treatment with other agents
- The dose is 375–500 mg/m$^2$ (maximum 1000 mg) intravenously at weeks 0 and 2, 50 mg/hr initially
- Premedication with methylprednisolone, antihistamine, and acetaminophen is recommended
- Adverse effects include infusion reactions, and progressive multifocal leukencephalopathy
- Improvement should be seen within 1 month of first infusion
- B cell counts should be checked before and 1 month after infusion
- Quantitative immunoglobulins should be checked every 3 months

## Prognosis
- Most studies that have evaluated long term outcomes of JIA done in the pre-biologic era
- Persistent oligoarticular JIA has generally the best outcome, with up to 50% of children achieving long-term remission, and <5% with moderate to severe limitation of function

- One third of those with oligoarticular JIA have an extended course over time
- Systemic JIA and RF-positive polyarticular JIA often have the worst prognosis, with up to 20% reporting moderate to severe limitation of function
- Fewer than 10% of children with RF-positive JIA achieve long-term remission
- It is unusual for children with JIA diagnosed in the recent years to end up in wheelchairs or need to use crutches for the most part
- With more aggressive therapy, use of DMARDs earlier, and the use of biological response modifiers, the long-term outcome is anticipated to improve for the next generation of children with JIA

## Pediatric systemic lupus erythematosus (pSLE)

Approximately 15–20% of all patients with SLE are diagnosed in childhood. The mean age of onset of pSLE is 12–14 years and it is rarely diagnosed before the age of 5. In contrast to adult SLE, at least 20% of patients are male. Discoid lupus erythematosus is less common in pediatric patients. Although the disease process is similar to that of adult-onset SLE, direct comparisons with pSLE are confounded by growth, development, and medication adherence issues. Overall, pSLE is associated with more aggressive disease activity, as children with SLE have a higher incidence of renal, hematologic, and neurologic involvement.

### Epidemiology
- pSLE is the second most common disease encountered in pediatric rheumatology clinics, while JIA is the most common
- The incidence rates for pSLE range from 0.36–2.5 per 100,000 children-years
- There is wide variation in prevalence of pSLE in the literature, ranging from 1.89–25.7 per 100,000 children
- Females are affected more than males
  - In younger children the female-to-male ratio is approximately 4:3
  - During the second decade of life the female-to-male ratio is 4:1

### Diagnosis
- The American College of Rheumatology classification criteria are useful in pSLE, although they are not diagnostic criteria and are validated only in adults

- Pediatric patients often present with constitutional symptoms, including fever, weight loss, and malaise
- Prepubertal children present more often with renal disease and hemolytic anemia, while postpubertal patients present with musculoskeletal and cutaneous features
- At least half of patients with pSLE have hematologic involvement at presentation
- Similar to adults, pSLE is associated with anti-dsDNA, anti-Smith, anti-RNP, anti-SSA(Ro), and anti-SSB(La)

## Disease course

- Over time patients with pSLE have more active disease compared to adults
- Studies have suggested that pSLE compared to adults is:
  - **More often** associated with renal disease, encephalopathy, chilblains, cutaneous vasculitis, malar rash, hemolytic anemia, leukopenia
  - **Less often** associated with discoid rash, arthralgias, myalgias, and sicca symptoms
    - <5% of isolated discoid lupus are encountered in patients under 15 years
- Race, ethnicity, and environmental influences are likely related to variations in disease expression over time
- Table 7.1 shows comparison of organ involvement in pSLE and adult SLE

## Management

- General
  - Psychosocial support is important
    - Assist with school issues and resources for children
  - Sun protection (sunscreen, sun avoidance, sun-protective clothing)
  - Growth
    - Growth failure occurs in approximately 15% of children
    - Puberty may be delayed
    - Although not well investigated, growth hormone may be associated with an increased risk of lupus flare
  - Bone health
    - 50% of bone mass is accrued during adolescence
    - Encourage exercise to promote bone density
    - Calcium and vitamin D
      - → Prepubertal children should receive 1000mg/day of calcium and postpubertal children should receive 1300–1500mg/day of calcium

**Table 7.1** Comparison of organ involvement in pSLE and adult SLE.

| Organ/tissue | pSLE | Adult SLE |
|---|---|---|
| Musculoskeletal | Trend toward more overt arthritis (non-erosive) and tenosynovitis<br>More than 90% of children who develop arthritis have presentation of joint symptoms within first year of disease<br>40% of children have osteopenia (defined as a Z score ≤-1)<br>6–10% of children have fractures related to osteopenia | Myalgias more common<br>Jaccoud arthropathy<br>Drug-induced myopathy<br>Among premenopausal adult women, 40% have osteopenia and 5% have osteoporosis |
| Mucocutaneous | Malar rash more frequent<br>60–80% of children have skin involvement at diagnosis<br>Raynaud phenomenon is seen in 15–20% of children | Photosensitivity and discoid lesions more frequent<br>Subacute cutaneous lupus more common<br>Raynaud phenomenon is seen in 20–40% of adults |
| Renal | Lupus nephritis (LN) often presenting feature<br>Up to 70% of children develop LN<br>Approximately 40% of children with LN develop hypertension<br>Proteinuria and urinary sediment abnormalities more common<br>5–10% of children with proliferative LN progress to end-stage renal disease within 5–10 years | LN affects 30–50% of adults<br>Studies vary on renal survival rates in adults, depending on WHO class, race, presence of hypertension, and age at onset, 5 year renal survival rate ranges from 50–95% |

(Continued)

**Table 7.1** *Continued*

| Organ/tissue | pSLE | Adult SLE |
|---|---|---|
| Neuropsychiatric (NPSLE) | Large variation in reports of children affected with NPSLE, but occurence at least as common as in adults<br><br>Within the 1st year of diagnosis, 70% of children develop NPSLE features<br><br>Most common mood disorder is depression<br><br>Cerebrovascular disease has been reported in up to 25% of pediatric patients<br><br>Cerebral vein thrombosis occurs in 15–25% of children, particularly lupus anticoagulant-positive patients<br><br>More children develop encephalopathy<br><br>Standardized assessments are being developed and validated in children | Cranial nerve abnormalities more common<br><br>Within the 1st year of diagnosis, approximately 30% develop NPSLE features |
| Hematologic | Almost all children develop hematologic involvement<br><br>Anemia of chronic disease is most common anemia<br><br>Hemolytic anemia is more prevalent in pediatric patients<br><br>Up to three quarters of children develop leukopenia<br><br>Neutropenia occurs in up to 15% of children<br><br>Overall, thrombocytopenia is more prevalent in children | Up to 80% of adults develop hematologic involvement<br><br>Similarly, anemia of chronic disease is most common anemia<br><br>Up to one quarter of adults develop leukopenia<br><br>Neutropenia occurs in up to 20% of adults |

| | | |
|---|---|---|
| Antiphospholipid antibody syndrome (APS) | Anti-phospholipid antibodies and/or lupus anticoagulant occur in 30–50% of patients<br>Children with the presence of lupus anticoagulant have 28-fold increased risk of thrombosis compared to children that persistently tested negative | Similarly, up to 50% of adults develop antiphospholipid antibodies and/or lupus anticoagulant<br>Development of APS is more common in adults |
| Cardiovascular | Pericarditis with pericardial effusion most common<br>Myocarditis, endocarditis, and conduction system abnormalities less common<br>In contrast to adults, transthoracic echocardiograms are often sufficient to diagnose Libman-Sacks disease<br>Premature atherosclerosis is a concern, although studies supporting the use of statins is lacking | Up to half of patients have evidence of pericardial thickening and/or effusion<br>Myocardial dysfunction has been reported in 5–60% of adults<br>Depending on the definition of abnormality, conduction defects affect 10 to 75% of adults<br>Increased risk of premature atherosclerotic disease among premenopausal women |
| Pulmonary | Involvement occurs in 25–75% of children<br>Wide range of manifestations from asymptomatic to life-threatening disease<br>Pleuritis most common<br>Chronic interstitial lung disease and pulmonary hypertension are rare | Involvement occurs in up to 90% of adults<br>Pleuritis most common<br>3–15% have chronic interstitial lung disease<br>5–15% have mild subclinical pulmonary hypertension |
| Gastrointestinal (GI) | Approximately 20% have GI involvement<br>Younger children are more susceptible<br>Although uncommon, pancreatitis may be present at diagnosis<br>Splenomegaly occurs in 20–30%<br>Hepatomegaly occurs in 40–50% | GI involvement varies depending on the definition of manifestation, but may occur in up to 70%<br>Hepatomegaly occurs in 10–30% |

→ Children should receive 600–1000 units/day of vitamin D
  ○ Intermittently monitor 25-hydroxy vitamin D levels and adjust dose (maximum of 5000 units/day)
- Dual-energy X-ray absorptiometry (DXA)
  → Precise use is in evolution
  → Recent pediatric reference data sets have been published for bone density measurements in children
  → Z scores of total body, lumbar spine, total hip, and femur may provide some indication of bone density
  → T scores are not useful in children, as they pertain to mean bone mineral density (BMD) at age 30, and should not be applied to growing children
  ○ Vaccinations
- Generally recommended, with the exception of live viral vaccines during times of active disease or while on immunosuppression
- Pneumococcal, meningococcal, *Haemophilus influenzae* type B, and annual inactivated influenza vaccine are recommended
  ○ Provide counseling regarding sexually transmitted disease, pregnancy, and contraception
  ○ Review risk factors for cardiovascular disease
  ○ Non-adherence is common and should be considered if a child is experiencing a lupus flare
- Medications
  ○ **Corticosteroids**
- Cornerstone of treatment
- Optimal dose and route have not been defined
  → Oral prednisone up to 2 mg/kg/day
  → Intravenous methylprednisolone pulse 30 mg/kg/dose (to maximum of 1000 mg)
- Comparisons of adult SLE and pSLE suggest that children are more often prescribed prednisone and receive intravenous methylprednisolone more frequently
  ○ **Antimalarials**
- Similar to adult SLE, most children receive hydroxychloroquine
  → 5–7 mg/kg/day
  → Emphasize the importance of routine ophthalmologic evaluation
- Chloroquine is rarely prescribed
  ○ **Azathioprine**
- Dose of 2–3 mg/kg/day
- Consider thiopurine methyltransferase testing prior to initiation

○ **Mycophenolate mofetil**
  ▪ $600 \, mg/m^2/dose$ twice per day (maximum of $3 \, g/day$)
  ▪ In contrast to adults, there are no randomized controlled trials of mycophenolate in pSLE
○ **Cyclophosphamide**
  ▪ Monthly pulse therapy of $500-1000 \, mg/m^2/dose$ used for lupus nephritis, neuropsychiatric lupus, or severe life-threatening manifestations
  ▪ Safety and efficacy of gonadotropin releasing hormone agonists for ovarian preservation has not been established in pSLE
○ B cell depleting therapy
  ▪ Case reports of benefit of **rituximab** in pSLE, particularly for refractory hemolytic anemia and thrombocytopenia
  ▪ Ongoing trial of belimumab in pSLE
  ▪ Identifying the developmental stages of B cells in pSLE versus adult SLE may enhance therapies in the future

## Prognosis

• Overall the prognosis has improved in recent years, but compared to adults, disease control and damage are poorer in children
  ○ In the 1950s, 5-year survival was 30–40%
  ○ In the 1980s, 5-year survival improved to >90%
  ○ Data from the University of California Lupus Outcomes Study (LOS) examined a cohort of patients with childhood-onset disease and found that 12% had died during the first 5 years of the study follow-up period
• Survival rates in children are associated with socioeconomic status, access to health care, educational background, ethnic background, infection, and active disease
• Children with renal or CNS involvement have increased mortality
• Morbidity due to lupus damage remains extensive
  ○ In a nested case–control study within the LUMINA (Lupus in MInorities, NAture versus nurture) trial, patients diagnosed during adolescence had a trend toward increased musculoskeletal and neuropsychiatric damage, while adult-onset disease trended toward more diabetes and peripheral vascular damage
  ○ In the LOS childhood-onset disease cohort, at the time of follow-up 68% of patients reported active disease

## Juvenile dermatomyositis

Juvenile dermatomyositis (JDM) is the most common inflammatory myopathy of childhood, compromising 85% of childhood-onset inflammatory myopathies. Juvenile polymyositis and overlap syndromes represent 8% and 7%, respectively, of the remaining 15% of patients. Inclusion body myositis is extremely rare in childhood. JDM is characterized by a systemic vasculopathy, manifesting as proximal muscle weakness and typical cutaneous features, which include heliotrope rash and Gottron's papules over the extensor surfaces of joints. In contrast to adult DM, children do not have an increased risk of malignancy and are less likely to develop interstitial lung disease.

### Epidemiology
• Incidence is 3.2 million cases per children per year in the United States
• More common in girls (2.3:1 female:male)
• Average age of onset is 7 years of age
• 25% of children are age 4 years or younger at disease onset
• No specific agents have been identified as triggers of JDM; although speculation about the role of infections has been suggested, no infectious agents have been confirmed in tissue or serum from patients to date

### Diagnosis
• Diagnostic criteria described by Peter and Bohan in 1975, although designed for adult inflammatory myopathy, can be applied to children with caution
  ○ More than 20% of children do not have elevation of creatinine kinase at diagnosis; thus, other myositis-associated enzymes (lactate dehydrogenase, aldolase, and transaminases) should be assayed
  ○ Patients with characteristic rash and two other criteria are considered to have probable JDM
  ○ Patients with characteristic rash and three other criteria are considered to have definite JDM
  ○ Pediatric rheumatologists less commonly use electromyography as a diagnostic tool
  ○ MRI via T2-weighted fat-suppressed or short tau inversion recovery (STIR) imaging is a sensitive technique for demonstrating muscle inflammation, although not specific for JDM

○ Nailfold capillaroscopy can distinguish JDM from muscular dystrophies, but does not differentiate JDM from other autoimmune connective tissue diseases, such as overlap myositis or mixed connective tissue disease

• The development of updated classification and diagnostic criteria for juvenile inflammatory myopathies is currently ongoing

## Etiology and pathogenesis

• JDM is a vasculopathy characterized histologically by capillary endothelial changes with lumen obliteration, perifasicular atrophy, perivascular inflammation, muscle fiber necrosis and regeneration, and tuboreticular inclusion bodies

• JDM is felt to occur in genetically susceptible hosts as the result of an unknown environmental trigger

○ Although infectious agents have been sought as an etiology, no direct association has been established

○ There has been some suggestion that birth seasonality may play a role, particularly in Hispanic individuals, but this has not been reproduced in other studies

• Cellular and humoral immunity contribute to the pathogenesis, and likely innate immunity as well

○ Dendritic cells appear to have a particularly important role

• More recently the role of interferon has been recognized, as gene expression profiles from affected muscle demonstrate upregulation of type-1 interferon genes

• Possible role for maternal microchimerism, as children with JDM have more maternally derived chimeric cells compared to healthy controls or siblings

• Role of myositis autoantibodies in juvenile myositis remains unknown

○ Anti-synthetase found in 5–10% of juvenile myositis

○ Anti-Mi2 found in 5% of juvenile myositis

○ Anti-SRP is rarely encountered in juvenile myositis

○ More recently, anti-p155 has been studied in JDM and was present in up to 30% of patients, although the clinical significance is uncertain

• A scoring system for JDM muscle biopsies has been developed by an international consensus working group based on the following domains:

○ Endomysial, perivascular, and perimysial inflammation

○ Vascular changes

○ Muscle fiber changes, including enhanced expression of MHC class I, perifasicular and muscle fiber atrophy, presence of neonatal myosin

○ Perimysial and endomysial fibrosis

## Disease course

- Four clinical phases:
  1) Prodrome
  2) Progressive rash and muscle weakness
  3) Persistent rash, weakness, and active myositis
  4) Recovery
- Disease course may be as short as 8 months, but may last for years in other patients
- Calcinosis
  - More prominent in JDM as compared to adult DM (Table 7.2)
  - Composed of calcium hydroxyapatite or carbonate apatite, but distinct from bone as specimens lack formal matrix seen in bone
  - Pressure points (elbows, knees, digits, and buttocks) are most commonly affected areas
  - Typically occurs 1–3 years after disease onset, but may be present at diagnosis or as much as 20 years later
  - Risk factors:
    - TNFα-308 polymorphism and increased production of TNFα
    - Delay in diagnosis
    - Inadequate treatment
    - Chronic disease course

**Table 7.2** System involvement in JDM compared to adult DM.

| Feature | % JDM | % Adult DM |
|---|---|---|
| Muscle weakness | 90–100 | 90–95 |
| Skin lesions | 90–100 | 70–90 |
| Gottron's papules | 60–90 | 50–60 |
| Heliotrope rash | 70–85 | 75 |
| Facial/malar rash | 40–80 | Data n/a |
| Periungal capillary changes | 80 | 40–50 |
| Ulcerations | 20–30 | 5–15 |
| Calcinosis | 20–30 | 5 |
| Arthritis/arthralgias | 30–60 | 50–70 |
| Fever | 15–45 | Data n/a |
| Joint contractures | 20–30 | Data n/a |
| Raynaud phenomenon | 5–15 | 10 |
| Gastrointestinal | 10–20 | 5–30 |
| Interstitial lung disease | 5 | 30–40 |
| Cardiac | <5 | 10–70 |
| Malignancy | Few case reports | 15–25 |

- ○ No established effective treatment
  - ▪ Colchicine, bisphosphonates, calcium-channel blockers, and bio-logics have been used
- ○ Surgery is reserved for patients with functional limitation, chronic pain, or recurrent infections at sites of calcinosis
- Lipodystrophy
  - ○ Occurs in 10–40% of patients
  - ○ May be focal, partial, or generalized
  - ○ Characterized by a gradual loss of subcutaneous and visceral fat, particularly over the face and upper body
  - ○ Typically occurs several years after disease onset
  - ○ Associated with insulin resistance, hypertriglyceridemia, hypertension, non-alcoholic steatohepatitis, and menstrual irregularities
  - ○ Therapy is not well defined

## Management

- General
  - ○ Photoprotection
  - ○ Physical therapy
  - ○ If there is evidence of esophageal dysmotility, involvement of speech therapy for appropriate swallowing precautions and safe feeding guidelines
  - ○ Calcium and vitamin D supplementation, particularly while on corticosteroids
    - ▪ Studies of children with JDM demonstrate decreased bone mineral density at diagnosis before exposure to corticosteroids
- Medications
  - ○ No randomized, controlled studies in children
  - ○ High-dose **corticosteroids** is standard therapy
    - ▪ No consensus on route
    - ▪ IV pulse methylprednisolone 30 mg/kg (up to 1000 mg) versus daily oral prednisone up to 2 mg/kg/day
  - ○ **Methotrexate**
    - ▪ Most often initiated at diagnosis with corticosteroids as a steroid-sparing agent, as reports have suggested that children may receive half the cumulative corticosteroid dose
    - ▪ 1 mg/kg or 15 mg/m$^2$
    - ▪ Oral or subcutaneous administration
  - ○ Second-line therapies
    - ▪ Intravenous immunoglobulin 2 g/kg monthly
    - ▪ Hydroxychloroquine

- Cyclosporine
- Mycophenolate mofetil
- Tacrolimus
- Azathioprine
- Rituximab
  - For severe or life-threatening disease
    - Cyclophosphamide
    - Bone marrow or stem cell transplant
  - The role of other biologics remains unclear
  - Although little data exists regarding treatment, consensus protocols for moderate JDM based on expert pediatric rheumatologists' input have been recently developed by the Childhood Arthritis and Rheumatology Research Alliance (CARRA) organization

## Prognosis

- Approximately one third of patients have a unicyclic course, while two thirds will have a polycyclic course or chronic persistent disease
- Risk factors for a poorer prognosis include:
  - Persistence of rash 6 months after diagnosis
  - Cutaneous ulcerations
  - Extensive calcinosis
  - Dysphagia or dysphonia
  - High serum creatinine kinase
  - Non-inflammatory vasculopathy on muscle biopsy
  - Advanced nail fold capillary changes
  - Delayed or inadequate treatment
- Prior to the recognition of the importance of corticosteroids in the treatment of JDM, mortality approached 40%, and has declined to <2% with current treatments

## Childhood vasculitis

Vasculitides are a complex group of diseases that may induce acute and chronic symptoms in both adults and children. Many childhood vasculitides share manifestations of the same disease in adults. However, some are much more prevalent in children and others may have unique features in young patients. This chapter will focus on the two most prevalent forms of vasculitis in childhood, Henoch Schönlein purpura (HSP) and Kawasaki disease (KD) and will highlight some unique features of granulomatosis with polyangiitis (GPA; Wegener's granulomatosis) in adolescents.

The incidence of vasculitis in individuals <17 years is 23 per 100,000. Of these: 49% are HSP and 23% KD; GPA accounts for only 4–8% of patients. HSP, sometimes termed anaphylactoid purpura, represents a vasculitis of small vessels and capillaries, whereas KD represents a medium-sized vessel vasculitis.

## Henoch Schönlein purpura
### Epidemiology
• HSP is more common in white individuals than in African-American individuals by 2:1
• HSP is more common in males than in females by 2:1
• Genetic factors, such as complement deficiencies and hereditary fever syndromes, may predispose to HSP
• Seasonal peaks in winter and spring suggest environmental factors, which may include:
  ○ Group A *Streptococcus*
  ○ *Staphylococcus aureus*
  ○ Influenza
  ○ Parainfluenza
  ○ EB virus
  ○ *Mycoplasma*
  ○ Ingested foods
  ○ Antibiotics (penicillin, ampicillin, erythromycin)
  ○ Vaccines (measles, typhoid, yellow fever)

### Etiology
• HSP is an IgA immune complex-mediated small vessel vasculitis

### Pathology
• Leukocytoclastic vasculitis primarily involving post-capillary venules with deposition of IgA immune complexes in vessel walls
• The glomerular histopathology is indistinguishable from IgA nephropathy (Berger's disease)

### Clinical features
• Skin
  ○ Purpura and petechiae with lower limb predominance, may present as target-like lesions and occasionally may be bullous
  ○ Lesions may involve arms, face, and ears
  ○ In children <1 year old, lesions are more diffuse and scalp edema may be seen

- Joints
  - Arthritis is common, affecting 75% of children
  - It is oligoarticular, non-erosive and self-limited
  - It may precede the rash in 25% of patients
- Gastrointestinal (GI)
  - Manifestations present in 50% of children and include colicky abdominal pain and occasional GI bleeding
  - Intussusception is an urgent complication seen in 2–4% of cases
  - GI manifestations may precede the rash in 25% of patients, sometimes leading to surgery for an acute abdomen
- Genitourinary
  - Manifestations present in 25–50% of children of which the most common is microscopic hematuria
  - Proteinuria may also occur and higher levels of protein loss are associated with a higher risk of long-term renal impairment which occurs in 2–15% of cases, whereas end-stage renal disease is rare (<1%)
  - Scrotal edema is also common and can mimic testicular torsion at times
- Other
  - Edema of hands, feet, and the periorbital region, irritability, and, rarely, seizures and stroke
  - Another rare but life-threatening complication is pulmonary hemorrhage

## Laboratory features
- Platelets normal or slightly increased
- ESR slightly increased
- IgA increased in 30%
- ANA negative

## Duration
- Duration is 4–6 weeks
- Recurrences are common (up to 40%) and usually occur in the first 6 months

## Treatment
- Generally supportive with NSAIDs and antacids
- Corticosteroid use has been controversial
  - They are used judiciously for severe GI and scrotal manifestations and for pulmonary and CNS manifestations
  - In a prospective study there was no evidence that corticosteroids prevented the development or progression of nephritis in HSP

## Kawasaki disease

- KD is the second most common childhood vasculitis, accounting for 23% of all childhood vasculitides
- When first reported in 1967 by Tomisaku Kawasaki it was termed mucocutaneous lymph node syndrome, which is a helpful way to remember its salient features
- It affects medium-sized vessels with a predilection for the coronary arteries

---

### EULAR/PreS classification criteria for Kawasaki disease

Fever that persists for ≥5 days + at least four of the following:
1. Bilateral conjunctival injection
2. Changes of the lips and oral cavity
   - Strawberry tongue
   - Diffuse redness of oropharyngeal mucosa
   - Erythema or cracking of lips
3. Cervical lymphadenopathy (>1.5 cm, usually unilateral)
4. Polymorphous exanthem
5. Changes in the peripheral extremities or perineal area
   - Erythema or edema of the palms or soles
   - Periungual desquamation in the subacute phase

Adapted from Ozen S, Pistorio A, Iusan SM, et al. (2010) *Ann Rheum Dis* 69:798–806.

---

### Epidemiology

- KD occurs most commonly in children <5 years of age
- 1.5 times more common in males than females
- Incidence in US 21 per 100,000; in Japan 219 per 100,000
- Manifestations in the very young (<6 months) or in older children and adolescents are often incomplete or atypical

### Etiology

- The cause is unknown
- It is thought to result from a hyper-activation of the immune system by an unknown infectious trigger in a genetically susceptible host

• Features of early age of onset, seasonality, and community outbreaks suggest an infectious cause; whereas, differences in ethnic incidence suggest a genetic predisposition
　○ For example, children born in the US of Japanese immigrants have four times the incidence of KD compared with white children
• There are theories that a superantigen leads to massive T lymphocyte activation, others have speculated that the presence of IgA plasma cells in the walls of coronary artery aneurysms suggest an oligoclonal IgA response
• Recent genetic studies have found an association with polymorphisms in the inositol 1,4,5-triphosphate 3-kinase C (ITPKC) gene that functions to downregulate T cell activation

## Pathology
• T lymphocyte infiltrates in the wall of small vessels, predominantly coronary arteries, leading to fusiform or saccular aneurysms, intimal proliferation, and thrombosis
• As noted above IgA plasma cells may also be seen

## Clinical features
• The features of Kawasaki disease present in three phases:
　○ **Active phase** – 10 days–2 weeks
　○ **Subacute phase** – 2–4 weeks; marked by thrombocytosis and periungual desquamation
　○ **Convalescent phase** – 4–8 weeks; marked by a normalization of the ESR and platelet count
• See the criteria for the diagnostic clinical features (Box)
• Coronary artery aneurysms (CAA) occur in ~20 % of untreated patients and in ~4% of treated patients
　○ Factors that increase risk of CAA are:
　　▪ Male gender
　　▪ Extremes of age
　　▪ Prolonged fever or fever after treatment
　　▪ Delay in diagnosis
　○ Two-dimensional (2-D) echocardiograms are recommended at diagnosis, at 2 weeks and between 6 and 8 weeks of diagnosis
• Other features
　○ Irritability
　○ Aseptic meningitis
　○ Hepatic dysfunction
　○ Hydrops of the gall bladder
　○ Sterile pyuria

---

**Kawasaki disease clinical pearls**

- Conjunctival injection is non-exudative with limbic sparing; a slit lamp exam will often reveal uveitis
- Cervical lymphadenopathy is one of the least common presenting signs
- There are no oral ulcers associated with KD
- Perianal and genital desquamation may precede periungual desquamation and can be seen as early as 3 days
- Testicular swelling and epididymitis may be seen
- Intravenous immunoglobulin (IVIG) will cause an elevation in the ESR, making this lab test a poor index of inflammation after treatment

---

- Incomplete Kawasaki disease
  - ○ These are patients who have 5 days of fever and only two or three of the other diagnostic features at presentation
  - ○ With the appropriate clinical features and supporting laboratory evidence, incomplete KD should be considered especially in patients at the extremes of age (<6 months or >9 years)
  - ○ Echocardiograms should be considered early in the evaluation of such patients

## Differential diagnosis
- Infections
  - ○ Viral, including measles, adenovirus, EBV, enterovirus, influenza
  - ○ Bacterial, including cervical adenitis, scarlet fever, staph scalded skin syndrome, toxic shock syndrome, leptospirosis
  - ○ Rickettsial, Rocky Mountain spotted fever
- Immune-mediated
  - ○ Stevens–Johnson Syndrome, serum sickness, acute rheumatic fever, systemic onset JIA, SLE, and other vasculitides
- Hereditary auto-inflammatory syndromes, such as TRAPS (tumor necrosis factor-associated periodic syndrome), hyper IgD syndrome, and cryopirin-associated periodic syndromes

## Laboratory features
- Neutrophilia with a left shift
- Hypoalbuminemia
- Elevated ESR often >40 mm/hr
- Elevated CRP
- Normocytic anemia

- Thrombocytosis often greater than $10^6/\mu L$ peaking in the subacute phase
- Elevated transaminases
- Sterile pyuria
- In patients responding poorly to therapy, these lab findings support additional therapy:
  - ○ CRP >10 mg/dL
  - ○ Hemoglobin (Hgb) <10 g/dL
  - ○ Elevated LDH

## Treatment guidelines for KD as recommended by the American Heart Association

- Initial treatment:
  - ○ IVIG 2 g/kg as a single infusion over 12 hours +
  - ○ Aspirin orally 80–100 mg/kg in four divided doses daily until afebrile for 48–72 hours
  - ○ After afebrile for 48–72 hours, reduce aspirin dose to 3–5 mg/kg/day and continue for 6–8 weeks if echo normal; continue this dose over an extended period of time if echo is abnormal
- Treatment after IVIG failure
  - ○ Treat with another dose of IVIG at 2 g/kg over 12 hours, if fever persists beyond 48 hours after completion of the initial dose of IVIG
- If there is no response to the second dose of IVIG:
  - ○ Give infliximab 5 mg/kg IV once, or
  - ○ Give methylprednisolone IV pulse therapy at 30 mg/kg daily for 1–3 days
- If there is still no response
  - ○ If methylprednisolone was given, give infliximab
  - ○ If infliximab was given, give cyclosporine A, methylprednisolone, or a second dose of infliximab
  - ○ Alternatively, give oral prednisone 1–2 mg/kg/day until the CRP is normal, then taper prednisone over 2 weeks
  - ○ Additional options include treatment with methotrexate or cyclophosphamide

### Keep in mind

Refractory disease and persistent fever increase the risk of coronary artery aneurysms.

## Granulomatosis with polyangiitis (GPA/Wegener's granulomatosis)

There are some unique features of this disease in childhood that warrant emphasis.

- In a study of 117 patients with antineutrophil cytoplasmic antibodies from the Childhood Arthritis and Rheumatology Research Alliance ARChiVe registry, 65 met ACR criteria for GPA
  - 63% were female
  - The median age was 14.2 years (range 4–17 years)
  - The median age from symptom onset to diagnosis was 2.7 months (range 0–49 months) (Cabral et al. 2009)
- Children with GPA have a higher risk of nasal deformity and subglottic stenosis than adults
- These features are incorporated into the Eular/PReS criteria (Box)

---

**EULAR/PReS Classification Criteria for childhood-onset GPA**

Diagnosis requires at least three of the following six features:
- Histopathological evidence of granulomatous inflammation
- Upper airway involvement
- Laryngo-tracheo-bronchial involvement
- Pulmonary involvement (by radiograph or CT)
- ANCA positivity
- Renal involvement (proteinuria, hematuria, RBC casts, necrotizing pauci-immune glomerulonephritis)

Adapted from Ozen S, Pistorio A, Iusan SM, et al. (2010) *Ann Rheum Dis* 69:798–806.

---

## Outcome measures in pediatric rheumatology

There are various instruments used to assess the outcomes of adults with rheumatologic diseases. Subjective and objective measures of disease activity, function and quality of life result in an improved evaluation of treatment and outcome. While some adult-based instruments are used in children, there are other tools designed specifically for the pediatric population. There is debate regarding the use of adult measures in children and efforts are being made to develop child-specific instruments.

## Validated measures in children

Common rheumatologic conditions of childhood include systemic lupus erythematosus, juvenile idiopathic arthritis, and juvenile dermatomyositis. See Table 7.3.

- Systemic lupus erythematosus (SLE)
  - ○ Systemic Lupus Erythematosus Disease Activity Index (SLEDAI)
    - The SLEDAI measures disease activity in **nine** organs/systems over the **last 10 days** looking at weighted, cumulative lupus disease activity
      - → Descriptors include seizure, psychosis, organic brain syndrome, visual disturbance, cranial nerve disorder, lupus headaches, CVA, vasculitis, arthritis, myositis, urinalysis findings (urinary casts, hematuria, proteinuria, pyuria), new rash, alopecia, mucosal ulcers, pleurisy, pericarditis, low complement, increased DNA binding, fever, thrombocytopenia, and leukopenia
    - Scores range from 0–105 points with higher scores indicating increased disease activity
    - Needs a complete history, physical exam, and laboratory results
    - This measure is also used in the adult population
  - ○ British Isles Lupus Assessment Group (BILAG)
    - The BILAG measures disease activity in single organs/individual systems
    - Encompasses **nine** systems over the **past 4 weeks in comparison to the previous 4 weeks**
      - → These systems include: general manifestations (i.e. fever, weight loss), mucocutaneous disease, CNS disease, renal disease, musculoskeletal disease, cardiovascular and respiratory disease, vasculitis, and hematological disease
    - Items are scored as 0 to 4, and then converted to alphabetical scores, grade A–E
      - → Grade A is very active disease needing immunosuppressive agents and/or steroids >20 mg or high-dose anticoagulation, and Grade E is no current or past disease activity
      - → This measure is also used in the adult population
  - ○ Systemic Lupus International Collaborating Clinics/American College of Rheumatology Damage Index (SLICC/SDI)
    - The SLICC/SDI measures permanent change or accumulated **damage** after SLE diagnosis in **12** organ systems for at **least 6 months**
      - → These include ocular, neuropsychiatric, renal, pulmonary, cardiovascular, peripheral vascular, gastrointestinal, musculoskeletal, skin, premature gonadal failure, diabetes, and malignancy

**Table 7.3** Common measures used in the evaluation of pediatric rheumatic diseases.

| Measures | Disease | Assessment | Patient or MD administered | Population |
|---|---|---|---|---|
| Childhood myositis assessment scale (CMAS) | Juvenile dermatomyositis | Evaluates muscle strength, physical function, and endurance in children with inflammatory myopathies | Patient or staff | Pediatric |
| Childhood Health Assessment Questionnaire (CHAQ) | Juvenile idiopathic arthritis | Evaluates physical function and the ability to perform activities of daily living | Self-report (patient and parent) | Pediatric |
| ACR20/50/70 | Juvenile idiopathic arthritis | Definition of improvement used in clinical trials in JIA | Patient and MD components | Pediatric |
| Systemic Lupus Erythematosus Disease Activity Index (SLEDAI) | Systemic lupus erythematosus | Measures disease activity over the past 10 days | MD administered | Pediatric Adult |
| British Isles Lupus Assessment Group (BILAG) | Systemic lupus erythematosus | Measures disease activity over the past 4 weeks | MD administered | Pediatric Adult |
| Systemic Lupus International Collaborating Clinics/American College of Rheumatology Damage Index (SLICC/SDI) | Systemic lupus erythematosus | Measures permanent change or accumulated damage after SLE diagnosis over at least 6 months | | |

- Scores range from 0–46, and damage is considered to occur if the score is ≥1
- This measure is also used in the adult population, but there is a **modified pediatric version available**
- Juvenile idiopathic arthritis (JIA)
  - Childhood Health Assessment Questionnaire (CHAQ)
    - The CHAQ was developed **specifically for children with JIA**
    - It is the most frequently used measure of **physical function** in pediatric rheumatology
    - Derived from the Stanford HAQ, which is a self-report questionnaire that also assesses physical function in activities of daily living in adults
    - There is a parent report and a child self-report for children ≥8 years of age
    - Evaluates physical function and the ability to perform activities of daily living in children 1–19 years of age
    - Contains 30 items in eight domains – dressing and grooming, arising, eating, walking, hygiene, reach, grip, and activities
    - Asks how much difficulty a child has in performing tasks over the past week
    - Scores range from 0–3 with higher scores indicating greater disability
    - Specific to pediatrics
  - ACR20/50/70 response
    - Definition of **improvement** used in clinical trials in JIA
    - Measures the improvement in **three** of any **six** core set variables by at least 20, 50, or 70%, respectively, without worsening of any single variable by more than 20, 50, or 70%
      - → Physician global assessment of disease activity (10 cm visual analog scale)
      - → Parent/patient global assessment of overall well-being (10 cm visual analog scale)
      - → Functional ability
      - → Number of joints with active arthritis
      - → Number of joints with limited range of motion
      - → ESR
    - Adult version includes seven core set variables – the six core set variables plus patient's assessment of pain
- Juvenile dermatomyositis (JDM)
  - Childhood Myositis Assessment Scale (CMAS)
    - The CMAS evaluates **muscle strength, physical function,** and **endurance** in children with inflammatory myopathies

- Focuses on upper and lower extremity muscle groups, but weighted toward lower extremity proximal and axial muscle groups
- A therapist-administered assessment that consists of 14 items wherein the activity is performed during CMAS administration
- Scores range from 0–52 with 52 indicative of normal or near-normal strength, function, or endurance; values less than 15 indicate severe disease
- Specific to pediatric population

## Further reading

### Juvenile idiopathic arthritis

Beukelman, T., Patkar, N.M., Saag, K.G., et al. (2011) American College of Rheumatology recommendations for the treatment of juvenile idiopathic arthritis: initiation and safety monitoring of therapeutic agents for the treatment of arthritis and systemic features. *Arthritis Care Res* (Hoboken) 63(4): 465–482.

Gowdie, P.J., Tse, S.M. (2012) Juvenile idiopathic arthritis. *Pediatric Cinics of North America* 59(2): 301–327.

Macaubas, C., Nguyen, K., Milojevic, D., Park, J.L., Mellins, E.D. (2009) Articular and polyarticular JIA: epidemiology and pathogenesis. *Nat Rev Rheumatol* 5(11): 616–626.

Petty, R.E., Southwood, T.R., Manners, P., Baum, J., Glass, D.N., Goldenberg, J., et al. (2004) International League of Associations for Rheumatology classification of juvenile idiopathic arthritis: second revision, Edmonton, 2001. *J Rheumatol* 31(2): 390–392.

Prahalad, S., Glass, D.N. (2008) A comprehensive review of the genetics of juvenile idiopathic arthritis. *Pediatr Rheumatol Online J* 6(1): 11.

Ravelli, A., Martini, A. (2007) Juvenile idiopathic arthritis. *Lancet* 369(9563): 767–778.

### Pediatric SLE

Brunner, H.I., Huggins, J., Klein-Gitelman, M.S. (2011) Pediatric SLE: towards a comprehensive management plan. *Nature Reviews Rheumatology* 7: 225–233.

Hersh, A., von Scheven, E., Yelin, E. (2011) Adult outcomes of childhood-onset rheumatic diseases. *Nature Reviews Rheumatology* 7: 290–305.

Levy, D.M., Kamphuis, S. (2012) Systemic lupus erythematosus in children and adolescents. *Pediatric Clinics of North America* 59: 345–364.

Mina, R., Brunner, H.I. (2010) Pediatric lupus: are there differences in presentation, genetics, response to therapy, and damage accrual compared to adult lupus? *Rheumatic Diseases Clinics of North America* 36: 53–80.

Silverman, E., Eddy, A. (2011) Systemic lupus erythematosus, in: Cassidy, J.T., Petty, R.E., Laxer, R.M., Lindsley, C.B. (Eds.), *Textbook of Pediatric Rheumatology*. Saunders, Philadelphia, PA.

### Juvenile dermatomyositis

Feldman, B.M., Rider, L.G., Reed, A.M., Pachman, L.M. (2008) Juvenile dermatomyositis and other idiopathic inflammatory myopathies of childhood. *Lancet* 371: 2201–2212.

Huber, A.M., Giannini, E., Bowyer, S.L., et al. (2010) Protocols for the initial treatment of moderately severe juvenile dermatomyositis: results of a Children's Arthritis and Rheumatology Research Alliance Consensus Conference. *Arthritis Care & Research* 62: 219–225.

Robinson, A.B., Reed, A.M. (2011) Clinical features, pathogenesis and treatment of juvenile and adult dermatomyositis. *Nature Reviews Rheumatology* 7: 664–675.

Ruperto, N., Pistorio, A., Ravelli, A., et al. (2010) The Paediatric Rheumatology International Trials Organisation provisional criteria for the evaluation of response to therapy in juvenile deramatomyositis. *Arthritis Care & Research* 62: 1533–1541.

## Childhood vasculitis

Cabral, D.A., Uribe, A.G., Benseler, S., et al. (2009) Classification, presentation, and initial treatment of Wegener's granulomatosis in childhood. *Arthritis and Rheumatism* 60: 3413–3424.

Newberger, J.W., Takahashi, M., Gerber, M.A., et al. (2004) Diagnosis, treatment, and long term management of Kawasaki disease. *Circulation* 110: 2747–2771.

Ozen, S., Pistorio, A., Iusan, S.M., et al. (2010) EULAR/PRINTO/PRES criteria for Henoch-Schönlein purpura, childhood polyarteritis nodosa, childhood Wegener's granulomatosis and childhood Takayasu arteritis: Ankara 2008. Part II: final classification criteria. *Annals of the Rheumatic Diseases* 69: 798–806.

Son, M.B., Gauvreau, K., Burns, J.C., et al. (2011) Inflixmab for immunoglobulin resistance in Kawasaki disease: a retrospective study. *Journal of Pediatrics* 158: 644–649.

Succimarri, R. (2012) Kawasaki disease. *Pediatric Clinics of North America* 59: 425–445.

Weiss, PF. (2012) Pediatric vasculitis. *Pediatric Clinics of North America* 59: 407–423.

## Pediatric outcome measures

Carle, A.C., Dewitt, E.M., Seid, M. (2011) Measures of health status and quality of life in juvenile rheumatoid arthritis: Pediatric Quality of Life Inventory (PedsQL) Rheumatology Module 3.0, Juvenile Arthritis Quality of Life Questionnaire (JAQQ), Paediatric Rheumatology Quality of Life Scale (PRQL), and Childhood Arthritis Health Profile (CAHP). *Arthritis Care & Research* 63(S11): S438–S445.

Giannini, E.H., Ruperto, N., Ravelli, A., et al. (2011) Preliminary definition of improvement in juvenile arthritis. *Arthritis and rheumatism.* 1997; 40(7): 1202–1209. Epub 1997/07/01.

Klepper SE. Measures of pediatric function: Child Health Assessment Questionnaire (C-HAQ), Juvenile Arthritis Functional Assessment Scale (JAFAS), Pediatric Outcomes Data Collection Instrument (PODCI), and Activities Scale for Kids (ASK). *Arthritis Care & Research* 63(S11): S371–S382.

Lattanzi, B., Consolaro, A., Solari, N., et al. (2011) Measures of disease activity and damage in pediatric systemic lupus erythematosus: British Isles Lupus Assessment Group (BILAG), European Consensus Lupus Activity Measurement (ECLAM), Systemic Lupus Activity Measure (SLAM), Systemic Lupus Erythematosus Disease Activity Index (SLEDAI), Physician's Global Assessment of Disease Activity (MD Global), and Systemic Lupus International Collaborating Clinics/American College of Rheumatology Damage Index (SLICC/ACR DI; SDI). *Arthritis Care & Research* 63(S11): S112–S117.

Rider, L.G., Werth, V.P., Huber, A.M., et al. (2011) Measures of adult and juvenile dermatomyositis, polymyositis, and inclusion body myositis: Physician and Patient/Parent Global Activity, Manual Muscle Testing (MMT), Health Assessment Questionnaire (HAQ)/Childhood Health Assessment Questionnaire (C-HAQ), Childhood Myositis Assessment Scale (CMAS), Myositis Disease Activity Assessment Tool (MDAAT), Disease Activity Score (DAS), Short Form 36 (SF-36), Child Health Questionnaire (CHQ), Physician Global Damage, Myositis Damage Index (MDI), Quantitative Muscle Testing (QMT), Myositis Functional Index-2 (FI-2), Myositis Activities Profile (MAP), Inclusion Body Myositis Functional Rating Scale (IBMFRS), Cutaneous Dermatomyositis Disease Area and Severity Index (CDASI), Cutaneous Assessment Tool (CAT), Dermatomyositis Skin Severity Index (DSSI), Skindex, and Dermatology Life Quality Index (DLQI). *Arthritis Care & Research* 63(S11): S118–S157.

Romero-Diaz, J., Isenberg, D., Ramsey-Goldman, R. (2011) Measures of adult systemic lupus erythematosus: Updated Version of British Isles Lupus Assessment Group (BILAG 2004), European Consensus Lupus Activity Measurements (ECLAM), Systemic Lupus Activity Measure, Revised (SLAM-R), Systemic Lupus Activity Questionnaire for Population Studies (SLAQ), Systemic Lupus Erythematosus Disease Activity Index 2000 (SLEDAI-2K), and Systemic Lupus International Collaborating Clinics/American College of Rheumatology Damage Index (SDI). *Arthritis Care & Research* 63(S11): S37–S46.

## CHAPTER 8

# HIV and rheumatic diseases

## Karen Law

Emory University School of Medicine, Atlanta, GA, USA

## Introduction

The spectrum of rheumatic diseases in HIV-infected patients continues to develop. HIV infection itself may cause rheumatic symptoms such as arthralgias and myalgias, as well as positive serologies that may confound diagnosis. A basic understanding of how the prevalence of certain rheumatic diseases may change as a patient's HIV status evolves, as well as knowledge of more rare disease syndromes in HIV that may mimic or overlap with traditional rheumatic diseases, can aid in more accurate diagnosis and treatment.

## General principles

- Polyclonal B cell activation from chronic inflammation in HIV induces multiple autoantibodies
  - ○ 45% of HIV patients have polyclonal gammopathy
  - ○ 20% of HIV patients have low-titer RF and ANA positivity
  - ○ Up to 90% of patients with AIDS have IgG anticardiolipin antibody
  - ○ These autoantibodies are **rarely clinically significant**, and do not correlate with developing a particular rheumatic syndrome
- HIV+ patients will often have **atypical patterns of serologies** (i.e. low-titer ANA+, centromere, RNP, SSB+, all in the same patient)
- Many of these patients may be initially **misdiagnosed** as having rheumatic disease instead of HIV

*Rheumatology Board Review*, First Edition. Edited by Karen Law and Aliza Lipson.
© 2014 John Wiley & Sons, Inc. Published 2014 by John Wiley & Sons, Inc.

---

**Helpful hints**

- Double-stranded DNA and low complement are **rare** in HIV
- Only typical patterns of serologies in the appropriate clinical setting are suggestive of underlying autoimmune disease
- Additional studies (x-ray, EMG, muscle biopsy, physical exam maneuvers such as Schober's test, etc.) can be helpful, as **compatible objective findings are a must!**

---

## The spectrum of rheumatic disease in HIV

- SLE and rheumatoid arthritis are **CD4+ T cell-mediated rheumatic diseases**
  - Therefore as CD4 count goes down with progressive HIV infection, these diseases become quiet
  - It is rare for either disease to develop in HIV-infected individuals, especially if CD4 count is <200 cells/μL
  - Conversely, with HIV treatment and immune reconstitution, SLE and RA may develop or recur, and may be quite severe
- Psoriasis and psoriatic arthritis are **CD8+ T cell-mediated rheumatic diseases**
  - During the course of progressive HIV infection, CD8-driven processes tend to worsen, as the CD4/CD8 ratio evolves
  - Therefore psoriasis and psoriatic arthritis become more prevalent in HIV patients as their CD4 count drops, and can be quite severe
  - Often highly active antiretroviral therapy (HAART) and immune reconstitution alone are effective for either condition
  - Refractory skin and joint involvement may require methotrexate (MTX), sulfasalazine (SSZ), or a TNF inhibitor
  - Hydroxychloroquine is typically avoided as it can worsen psoriasis; additionally new data suggests it is associated with a **decline in CD4 cell count** and **increased viral replication** when used in HIV-infected patients not taking antiretroviral therapy

## Approach to evaluating joint pain in HIV

- HIV-associated arthralgias
  - Up to 45% of HIV-infected patients may have unexplained arthralgias
  - Many report arthralgias/myalgias as part of an HIV seroconversion syndrome

○ Some hypothesize a role of elevated circulating cytokines or transient bone ischemia in response to HIV infection
○ Patients with isolated arthralgia rarely progress to inflammatory joint disease
○ Primary treatments include non-narcotic analgesics and reassurance
○ Autoantibodies are sometimes difficult to interpret in this setting
• HIV-associated arthritis
  ○ Similar to a "seronegative rheumatoid arthritis"
  ○ Inflammation/synovitis is visible on exam
  ○ Usually an asymmetric oligoarthritis, primarily involving lower extremities
  ○ Self-limited, usually lasts <6 weeks
  ○ Some case reports of more chronic, erosive arthritis but this is rare
  ○ Treatment: NSAIDs, low-dose glucocorticoids in severe cases for a limited amount of time; plaquenil or SSZ also have been used

---

### Keep in mind

HIV-associated arthritis, in contrast to HIV-associated reactive arthritis (discussed below) is not associated with concomitant infection, and requires less intense treatment for a shorter course. It also does not typically result in contractures or erosions.

---

• HIV-associated reactive arthritis and spondyloarthropathy
  ○ HIV-associated reactive arthritis
    ▪ Asymmetric oligo- or polyarthritis with dactylitis
    ▪ Mucocutaneous involvement: keratoderma blenorrhagicum, circinate balanitis, uveitis, urethritis
    ▪ Enthesopathy is common
    ▪ Synovial fluid sometimes reveals microorganisms such as *Chlamydia*
    ▪ Associated with HLA-B27
    ▪ More common in HIV-infected patients, possibly due to coincidence of HIV and other sexually transmitted diseases (STDs) in high-risk populations; animal studies point to a pathogenic role of HIV infection
    ▪ Diagnosis indicated by typical musculoskeletal and skin findings; other helpful findings include **sacroiliitis** or **erosions** on plain films,

positive culture of a typical organism from urine or cervical swab, and inflammatory synovial fluid on arthrocentesis
- Treatment
  - → Similar to HIV-negative patients with reactive arthritis – NSAIDs, SSZ, MTX, and in some cases TNF inhibitors have been used with caution
- Undifferentiated spondyloarthropathy
  - Most common form of spondyloarthropathy in HIV
  - Mix of reactive arthritis, ankylosing spondylitis, psoriatic arthritis – no classic pattern and may be elusive to diagnose

---

**Keep in mind**

Traditionally spondyloarthropathies are RF negative, however they may be RF+ (false positive) in HIV patients due to polyclonal B cell activation from chronic inflammation

---

## HIV-associated syndromes that mimic/overlap rheumatic syndromes

- **DILS: diffuse idiopathic lymphocytic syndrome**
  - Limited to HIV+ patients
  - Characterized by >6 months of **massive** bilateral salivary gland enlargement or severe xerostomia
  - Extraglandular manifestations
    - Interstitial pneumonitis
    - Neurologic manifestations – cranial nerve (CN) palsy, aseptic meningitis, peripheral motor neuropathy
    - Transaminitis from CD8 infiltration into liver
    - Renal type IV RTA (renal tubular acidosis)
    - Also associated with polymyositis and lymphoma
  - Pathologic specimens show salivary or lacrimal gland CD8+ lymphocytic infiltration without granulomatous or neoplastic involvement
  - **Symptoms usually present within 3 years of HIV diagnosis; DILS is paradoxically associated with early HIV, higher CD4 count, and fewer opportunistic infections**

○ Treatment: HAART, steroids for glandular swelling, pilocarpine for sicca symptoms

○ **Differentiating DILS and Sjögrens syndrome** – Sjögren's syndrome has:

- Lesser degree of salivary gland swelling; less symmetric
- Lesser degree of lymphadenopathy
- **CD4 cell infiltration** (not CD8 as in DILS) on pathology
- Positive autoantibodies in a typical pattern – RF, SSA/B, ANA
- Steroids for glandular symptoms in Sjögren's are rarely helpful
- Interstitial lung disease, when present in Sjogren's syndrome, is typically asymptomatic

- **Macrophage activiation syndrome**
  ○ Also known as hemophagocytic lymphohistiocytosis
  ○ Reflects widespread immune dysregulation in response to varied triggers:
    - Rheumatic disease – Still's disease, SLE
    - Infection – HIV, EBV, hepatitis A, CMV, coxsackie, varicella, parvovirus
    - Malignancy – leukemia, lymphoma
  ○ T lymphocyte dysregulation results in proinflammatory cytokine overproduction and an unchecked immune response characterized by
    - Abnormal proliferation and regulation of macrophages
    - Consumptive coagulopathy
    - Deficient natural killer (NK) cell activity
    - Think of it like disseminated intravascular coagulation (DIC) of the immune system
  ○ Clinical manifestations:
    - Fever
    - Hepatosplenomegaly
    - Purpuric, non-blanching rash
    - Pancytopenia
    - Transaminitis
  ○ Patients progress to multiorgan dysfunction and DIC; mortality is high
  ○ Diagnosis may be difficult as many features are consistent with those of the causative underlying illness:
    - **Elevated ferritin >1000 μg/L**
    - **Elevated triglycerides**
    - Elevated soluble CD25, a subunit of IL2 that reflects T cell activation

- Elevated soluble CD163, a macrophage transmembrane protein reflecting macrophage activation
- Tissue demonstration of hemophagocytosis – usually by bone marrow biopsy

○ Successful diagnosis rests on **maintaining a high index of suspicion**, especially if a patient's disease course is worsening despite appropriate treatment for the underlying illness

○ Treatment – limited studies due to rarity of disease and heterogeneity of causative illnesses

- Early trials emphasize prompt recognition and initiation of pulse methylprednisolone
- Patients that do not respond to steroids may require etoposide, cyclosporine, or IVIG
- Anakinra offers a newer approach: theoretically it interrupts the proinflammatory cytokine cascade to terminate dysregulated T cell proliferation

- **HIVIC: HIV-associated immune complex glomerulonephritis with "lupus-like" features**

○ Patients present with sudden, severe renal insufficiency and proteinuria

○ Primarily in white and Asian patients

○ Renal biopsy shows immune complex glomerulonephritis, not focal segmental glomerulosclerosis (FSGS) or HIV-associated nephropathy (HIVAN) which is more typical of HIV nephropathy

- "Full house" pattern of immunofluorescence (IF) with positive staining for IgG, IgM, IgA, C3, and C1q which is classic for lupus nephritis
- Subendothelial and subepithelial immune complex deposits are present
- Wire loops
- Hyaline thrombi

○ Differentiating HIVIC from lupus nephritis

- Most patients with HIVIC lack other serologic or clinical evidence for SLE, and usually have low CD4 counts that would make SLE unlikely
- However, atypical patterns of autoimmune serologies may be seen due to immune dysregulation

○ Treatment of HIVIC

- **Correct diagnosis as HIVIC, not lupus nephritis is critical, as treatment strategies differ substantially**

- Therefore, all patients with a new diagnosis of SLE presenting with lupus nephritis **must be tested for HIV**
- Treatment of HIVIC is HAART and anticoagulation if proteinuria is severe
  - → Some case reports report improvement with steroids
  - → Renal survival is poor, and most progress to end-stage renal disease (ESRD)
  - → These patients should **not** be treated with traditional lupus nephritis protocols

## Further reading

Calabrese, L.H., Kirchner, E., Shrestha, R. (2005) Rheumatic complications of human immunodeficiency virus infection in the era of highly active antiretroviral therapy. *Seminars in Arthritis and Rheumatism* 35: 166–174.

Haas, M., Kaul, S., Eustace, J.A. (2005) HIV-associated immune complex glomerulonephritis with "lupus-like" features: a clinicopathologic study of 14 cases. *Kidney International* 67: 1381–1390.

Maganti, R.M., Reveille, J.D., Williams, F.M. (2008) Therapy Insight: the changing spectrum of rheumatic disease in HIV infection. *Nature Clinical Practice Rheumatology* 4(8): 428–438.

Nguyen, B.Y., Reveile, J.D. (2009) Rheumatic manifestations associated with HIV in the highly active antiretroviral therapy era. *Current Opinion in Rheumatology* 21: 404–410.

Tristano, A.G. (2008) Macrophage activation syndrome: a frequent but under-diagnosed complication associated with rheumatic diseases. *Medical Science Monitor* 14: RA27–36.

# CHAPTER 9

# Miscellaneous arthropathies

## Robin Geletka[1], Karen Law[2]

[1]Actelion Pharmaceuticals Ltd, San Francisco, CA, USA
[2]Emory University School of Medicine, Atlanta, GA, USA

## Introduction

Arthritis can often be a manifestation of underlying systemic disease. Arthritis from malignancy and hematologic disorders, endocrinopathies, and infectious disease must be considered in the differential list in patients presenting with arthritis. Understanding the characteristics of these disorders is critical to making the diagnosis of the underlying disease.

## Arthritis from malignancy and hematologic disorders

### Paraneoplastic syndromes
- May coincide with, follow, or precede onset of malignancy
- Treatment involves therapy directed towards primary malignancy
- **Hypertrophic osteoarthropathy**
  - Characterized by proliferation of bone at distal extremities
  - Associated with **clubbing, periosteal proliferation** of tubular bones, and joint effusions
  - May be associated with lung malignancy; in these cases resection of malignancy results in resolution of arthropathy
  - Synovial WBC count is non-inflammatory
  - Pain involves both joint and bone
- **Carcinomatous polyarthritis**
  - Inflammatory seronegative polyarthritis
  - Late age of onset and commonly **spares hands and wrists**

*Rheumatology Board Review*, First Edition. Edited by Karen Law and Aliza Lipson.

○ Typically there is no evidence of direct metastasis
○ Found more commonly in **women with breast cancer** and **men with lung cancer**
- **Erythromelalgia**
  ○ Intense **pain, redness**, and **warmth** in the digits, palms, and soles
  ○ Most commonly found in patients with polycythemia vera or essential thrombocytosis, though it may also be idiopathic
  ○ Responds to aspirin, dosed up to 650 mg TID

## Direct tumor invasion causing arthritis

- Leukemic arthritis
  ○ Most common in acute lymphocytic leukemia in children
  ○ Asymmetric polyarthritis of large joints
  ○ Severe joint and bone pain
  ○ Leukemic cells can be found in synovial fluid or synovial tissue
  ○ Associated with an increased frequency of gout and septic arthritis
- Lymphomatous arthritis
  ○ A rare mono- or polyarthritis
  ○ Affected patients also experience increased frequency of gout and septic arthritis
- Multiple myeloma
  ○ Malignant plasma cell tumor often associated with axial bone pain
  ○ Arthritis is rare
  ○ Associated with AL amyloid arthropathy
    ▪ Symmetric, non-inflammatory arthritis
    ▪ Typically affects shoulders, wrists, and knees
    ▪ Shoulder involvement is called "shoulder pad sign"
    ▪ Diagnosis made by bone marrow biopsy, presence of M protein, and biopsy of synovium showing amyloid
- Metastatic carcinomatous arthritis
  ○ Lung cancer is the most common cause
  ○ Manifests as a non-inflammatory monoarthritis of large joints

## Hematologic disorders

- Hemophilia A and B
  ○ **Recurrent hemarthrosis** is the most common manifestation
  ○ May occur spontaneously or following trauma
  ○ Over time, patients may develop a chronic arthropathy thought to be secondary to repeated bleeding episodes and deposition of iron in the synovium
  ○ Associated with **osteonecrosis (AVN) of the hip**

○ Treatment involves factor replacement, immobilizaton, and ice

○ Patients have a much higher risk of septic arthritis; a low threshold for joint aspiration is recommended if infection is suspected

- Sickle cell disease

○ Sickle cell arthropathy is caused by microvascular ischemia, usually in large joints

○ Associated with **osteonecrosis** most often affecting the hip

○ Vaso-occlusive crises may result in **dactylitis**, which may be the presenting symptom of sickle cell disease in children

## Endocrinopathies

Disorders of the endocrine system, or endocrinopathies, can be associated with musculoskeletal manifestations involving the joints, bone, tendons, nerves, and soft tissue. This section will go in to further detail about the musculoskeletal manifestations of endocrine disorders.

### Diabetes mellitus

- Diabetes mellitus is associated with a higher risk of multiple musculoskeletal manifestations, most of which are associated with poor glycemic control

- **Diabetic cheiroarthropathy**

○ A disorder involving the soft tissues of the hands and fingers resulting in waxy skin thickening and tightening and joint contractures

○ Classic finding called the **"prayer sign,"** in which the palms and fingers do not touch when the hands are pressed together

○ Pathogenesis is believed to be related to excess glycosylation of collagen in the skin and joint tissues

- **Adhesive capsulitis**

○ A condition causing limitation in shoulder motion often called "frozen shoulder"

○ Treatment can involve a combination of NSAIDs, steroid injections, and physical therapy

- **Dupuytren's contracture**

○ An abnormality of the collagen in the flexor tendons of the hand, causing shortening and nodularity

○ Patients affected have an inability to fully flex or extend affected fingers

○ Treatment includes surgical removal of collagen followed by physical therapy

○ Newer treatments involve local injection of a collagen-digesting enzyme, followed by physical therapy; though this technique avoids a surgical procedure, it is associated with a higher risk of tendon rupture

- **Flexor tenosynovitis**
  ○ Also known as "trigger finger"
  ○ Caused by thickening or nodularity of the flexor tendon
  ○ The thickened tendon glides abnormally, causing it to get "caught" at the A1 pulley at the metacarpal head
  ○ The result is a sticking sensation on flexion or extension that causes extreme pain when force is used to overcome the restriction
  ○ Unlike flexor tenosynovitis not associated with DM, those associated with DM respond poorly to local steroid injection and often recur, requiring surgical intervention for definitive treatment

- **Diabetic amyotrophy**
  ○ A condition which often causes muscle weakness resulting from a non-inflammatory mononeuropathy
  ○ Usually affects the thigh, hip, and buttocks
  ○ EMG can be used to suggest the condition and rule out other conditions

- **Diabetic muscle infarction**
  ○ Typically presents as acute, localized swelling and pain, usually in a lower extremity, that persists for several weeks
  ○ Creatine kinase (CK) may be elevated or normal
  ○ Other conditions such as infection and thrombosis must be ruled out
  ○ MRI can establish the diagnosis, but in the correct clinical setting is not necessary
  ○ Treatment is conservative, with pain management and activity restriction in the acute phase, followed by physical therapy in later stages

- Other DM-associated syndromes are discussed elsewhere in this text:
  ○ DISH
  ○ Neuropathic arthritis
  ○ Carpal tunnel syndrome

## Thyroid disease

- Hyperthyroidism
  ○ Thyroid acropachy
    ▪ An extreme manifestation of Graves disease
    ▪ Patients exhibit **soft tissue swelling** of hands, fingers, and toes with clubbing

- **Periostitis** is evident on x-ray
- Often associated with thyroid dermopathy and thyroid ophthalmopathy
  ○ Hyperthyroidism is also associated with a non-inflammatory proximal myopathy
    - Usually seen in the setting of toxic multinodular goiter or Graves disease
    - Caused by direct toxic effect of thyroxine on muscle fibers
    - Heat intolerance in addition to muscle fatigue can be a clue to the diagnosis that helps to exclude other diagnoses
    - CK is typically elevated, and thyroid tests suggest hyperthyroidism
- Hypothyroidism
  ○ Associated with a myopathy with elevated CK levels and compatible thyroid tests; therefore hypothyroid myopathy must be ruled out when evaluating for inflammatory myopathy
  ○ Non-inflammatory joint effusions and arthralgias are often seen
  ○ Can be associated with **pseudogout** or asymptomatic chondrocalcinosis

## Parathyroid disease: Hyperparathyroidism

- As with hypothyroidism, hyperparathyroidism can be associated with a non-inflammatory arthritis, as well as **pseudogout** and chondrocalcinosis
- Hyperparathyroidism is also associated with **osteopenia** and early **osteoporosis**
- **Osteitis fibrosa cystica** is a syndrome in which uncontrolled hyperparathyroidism induces excess bone breakdown, causing the bones to become soft, painful, and deformed
  ○ May be seen in primary hyperparathyroidism as well as **renal osteodystrophy**, or hyperparathyroidism associated with chronic kidney disease
  ○ X-rays show bone cysts and subperiosteal erosions, as well as thin bones and bowing
  ○ Erosions in the pelvis may mimic sacroiliitis, and must be interpreted in the appropriate clinical setting to arrive at the correct diagnosis

## Acromegaly

- Acromegaly is caused by abnormal increased secretion of growth hormone and its primary mediator, insulin-like growth factor (IGF) 1
- A wide spectrum of rheumatic diseases is common in acromegaly
- Manifestations include a non-inflammatory arthritis that can be quite disabling, due to early osteoarthritis and abnormal repair mechanisms

- Joints affected are primarily the knees, shoulders, and lumbosaral spine
- X-rays typically show **widened joint spaces** due to excess cartilage growth early on, followed by more typical findings of osteoarthritis
- Some patients also develop **DISH**, associated with the development of diabetes mellitus
- Premature osteoarthritis with carpal tunnel syndrome are commonly the initial signs of acromegaly
- Acromegaly can also be associated with pseudogout and chondrocalcinosis
- Bone changes are usually irreversible even once treatment begins

## Infectious arthritis

Arthritis is a serious manifestation of infectious diseases and carries significant morbidity and mortality. This section will go into detail about common presentations of arthritis associated with bacteria, viruses, mycobacteria, fungi, and syndromes associated with streptococci.

### Septic arthritis
- Non-gonococcal septic arthritis is the most common and most serious cause of septic arthritis
  - ○ Clinical presentation
    - Usually **monoarticular**; the knee is the most common joint involved
    - In a patient with acute monoarthritis, septic joint should always be ruled out with an arthrocentesis
    - Usually accompanied by fever or signs of infection elsewhere, unless the patient is immunocompromised
  - ○ Etiology
    - Gram-positive cocci cause most cases of septic arthritis with *Staphylococcus aureus* being the most common organism
    - Gram-negative bacilli are more common in those with underlying comorbidities
    - *S. epidermidis* occurs in prosthetic joints and may present many years after joint replacement
  - ○ Risk factors
    - Age >80 years
    - Diabetes mellitus
    - Prosthetic joints

- Rheumatoid arthritis
- Preceding skin infection
- Intravenous drug use
- Immunocompromise
- Chronic kidney or liver disease
○ Pathogenesis
  - Most common cause is hematogenous spread from an extra-articular site such as the skin or other site of infection
  - Direct inoculation is uncommon
  - Prosthetic joint infection may occur more than a year after surgery due to seeding at the time of surgery
  - Consider evaluating for **subacute bacterial endocarditis** if several joints are involved, or if the patient is bacteremic
○ Diagnosis
  - Arthrocentesis and synovial fluid analysis are the mainstay of diagnosis
    → Order cell count, gram stain/culture, and crystal analysis
    → Synovial fluid WBC is usually greater than 50,000/mm$^3$ with a predominance of PMNs
    → Gram stain is positive about 50% of time
  - Blood cultures are positive about 50% of time
  - If WBC count is greater than 100,000/mm$^3$, empiric treatment should begin for septic arthritis until cultures return

---

**Keep in mind**

Coexistence of infection and crystal disease such as gout or pseudogout can occur; therefore the presence of crystals on synovial fluid examination does not rule out the possibility of septic arthritis.

---

○ Treatment
  - Once septic arthritis is suspected, treatment should be initiated promptly after appropriate cultures are obtained
  - Antibiotic choice is based on clinical scenario and may be refined based on gram stain results and final culture results
  - Adequate drainage of the infected joint space must be achieved through either repeated needle aspirations or surgical wash-out, in consultation with orthopedic surgery
  - **Inadequate drainage can result in inability to clear the infection as well as long-term loss of joint function**

- Gonococcal septic arthritis requires specific considerations:
  - Caused by *Neisseria gonorrhea*
  - Occurs primarily in otherwise healthy young adults who are sexually active
  - Patients with **acquired or congenital complement deficiencies** are also high risk for gonococcal infections
  - Dissemminated gonococcal infection typically follows two patterns:
    - Constitutional symptoms, painless pustular dermatitis, migratory non-purulent arthritis, and tenosynovitis
    - Constitutional symptoms and purulent arthritis, without dermatitis
  - Synovial fluid gram stain and culture are usually negative unless the arthritis is purulent
  - Cultures at extra-articular sites such as rectum, throat, and genitourinary tract may aid in diagnosis
  - Treatment of choice is a third-generation cephalosporin with the addition of doxycycline or azithromycin due to emerging increased resistance; additionally, all sexual partners should be assessed and treated

## Viral arthritis

- **Parvovirus**
  - Acute self-limited disease caused by parvovirus B19 that mimics rheumatoid arthritis
  - Generally lasts less than 6 weeks
  - Typically involves contact with school-aged children or infected individuals
  - Diagnosed by positive B19 IgM antibodies; IgG antibodies are not sufficient for diagnosis and are indicative only of past exposure
  - Treatment is conservative with primarily NSAIDs and non-narcotic analgesics; in some instances a short course of low-dose prednisone provides symptomatic relief
- **Hepatitis C (HCV)**
  - May present as a non-erosive polyarthritis or polyarthralgias
  - Can mimic or coexist with rheumatoid arthritis, causing diagnostic uncertainty in some cases
  - Positive rheumatoid factor may exist in up to 50% of patients with HCV
  - **True rheumatoid arthritis patients typically exhibit positive rheumatoid factor, as well as antibodies to CCP, erosive disease, and synovitis**

○ HCV is also linked to type II cryoglobulinemia and cryoglobulinemic vasculitis, causing purpura over the lower extremitites, arthralgias, membranoproliferative glomerulonephritis, and ischemic necrosis

- **Hepatitis B (HBV)**
  ○ Acute HBV infection can be associated with a self-limited syndrome with inflammatory polyarthritis, fever, and skin rashes that may mimic rheumatoid arthritis
    ▪ Arthritis is generally self-limited and remits with the onset of jaundice
    ▪ HBV is also linked to **polyarteritis nodosa**, an ANCA-negative, necrotizing vasculitis of medium-sized arteries

- **Rubella**
  ○ Acute infection may cause a self-limited polyarthritis or polyarthrlagias with morning stiffness mimicking rheumatoid arthritis
  ○ Fever, facial rash, cervical lymphadenopathy, and conjunctivitis are distinguishing features
  ○ Postvaccination arthropathy has been described in the weeks following rubella vaccination and is generally benign and self-limited

## Mycobacterial infections and arthropathy

- Tuberculosis infection is associated with several different patterns of arthritis
  ○ Peripheral arthritis
    ▪ Typically occurs as chronic monoarthritis affecting the hip or knee
    ▪ Usually due to reactivation of latent TB; may not be associated with disease elsewhere and chest x-ray may be normal
    ▪ **Synovial biopsy** is the definitive diagnostic test whenever TB is suspected; synovial fluid is insensitive and may be normal on repeated aspirations
  ○ Spinal tuberculous arthritis
    ▪ Known as **Pott's disease**; it is the most common form of TB arthritis
    ▪ Typically occurs in thoracic vertebrae with infection starting in anterior portion of vertebral bodies
    ▪ Vertebral body collapse results in kyphosis and a characteristic gibbus formation, or sharp angle in the spinal curvature, seen on x-ray
  ○ **Poncet's disease**
    ▪ Sterile, reactive polyarthritis occurring during active TB
    ▪ Joint and tissue cultures are negative

- Erythema nodosum is a rare, but classic associated finding
- Initiation of antituberculous medications results in rapid resolution of symptoms

> Bacillus Calmette-Guerin exposure (BCG) has been associated with arthralgias and arthritis when used as either as a vaccine or as immunotherapy for bladder cancer.

- Arthropathies associated with atypical mycobacteria
  - Typically indolent, chronic infections that can involve bone, joint, tendon, or bursa
  - Most commonly affects hands and wrists
  - Generally transmitted via direct inoculation
  - Risk factors include trauma, surgery, and previous glucocorticoid use
  - *Mycobacterium marinum* is specifically associated with acquatic exposures such as lakes, fish tanks, etc.
  - Diagnosis is made by the presence of mycobacteria in synovial tissue or fluid, although, as with tuberculous mycobacteria, synovial fluid is notoriously insensitive

## Fungi
- **Candida**
  - A rare cause of arthritis that can be either indolent or acute
  - May be transmitted by direct inoculation or hematogenously
  - Risk factors include intravenous drug use, older age with comorbidities, and exposure to antibiotics, chemotherapy, or other immunosuppressive agents
  - Diagnosis rests on culture of synovial fluid
- **Histoplasmosis**
  - Endemic in the Ohio and Mississippi River Valleys
  - More prevalent in immunocompromised patients, or patients on glucocorticoids or TNF-alpha inhibitor therapies
  - Typically auses an immunologically mediated migratory polyarthritis associated with acute infection; true infection of the joint is rare
- **Coccidiomycosis**
  - Endemic in the southwestern US
  - Valley fever is a self-limited, immunologically mediated polyarthritis that occurs during acute infection

○ Typically associated with fever, rash, hilar adenopathy, and erythema nodosum

○ In rare instances, a chronic infectious arthritis can develop, usually involving the knees

- **Sporotrichosis**
  ○ Caused by the dimorphic fungus *Sporothrix schenckii*
  ○ Occurs through inoculation of organism into the skin through gardening or exposure to soil or plant material such as rose thorns
  ○ Most commonly causes a chronic monoarthritis with classic skin findings, including ulcerating papules that classically follow lymphatic channels
  ○ Diagnosed by fluid or tissue culture from a skin lesion

# CHAPTER 10

# Osteoporosis

## Karen Law

Emory University School of Medicine, Atlanta, GA, USA

## Introduction

Osteoporosis is a large-scale issue among the general population, affecting more than 10 million Americans. Osteoporosis-related fractures occur at a rate of 1.5 million/year in the US, and are a significant economic burden related to surgery, hospital stay, rehab, disability, and long-term care. Patients with rheumatic diseases are at increased risk of osteoporosis due to glucocorticoid and other medications, decreased activity, and decreased vitamin D.

## Diagnosis

- Patients who have suffered a fragility or insufficiency fracture have osteoporosis by definition, regardless of DEXA (dual energy x-ray absorptiometry) results
- DEXA is used to diagnose patients with osteoporosis before a fragility fracture is sustained
    - **Plain films are not appropriate for early screening of osteoporosis as 30% of bone mineral density is lost before this is apparent on x-ray!**
- WHO criteria for osteoporosis based on DEXA (Table 10.1)
    - Osteoporosis if T score is ≤ –2.5
    - Severe osteoporosis if T score is ≤ –2.5 and presence of fragility fracture
    - Osteopenia if T score is between –1 and –2.5
- Limitations of DEXA scanning
    - WHO criteria for osteoporosis are based on a postmenopausal, white female study population; applicability to other ethnic groups or males is unknown

*Rheumatology Board Review*, First Edition. Edited by Karen Law and Aliza Lipson.
© 2014 John Wiley & Sons, Inc. Published 2014 by John Wiley & Sons, Inc.

**Table 10.1** Interpreting DEXA scan results.

| Result | Clinical correlation |
| --- | --- |
| T score | Compares patient's BMD with peak bone mass in young normal subjects |
| Z score | Compares patient's BMD with BMD of age-matched subjects |
| Absolute BMD | Best for long-term individual follow-up and determining a patient's response to therapy |

**Table 10.2** Clinical risk factors assessed in FRAX.

Age
Sex
Current smoking
Alcohol intake
BMI
Previous fragility fracture
Previous glucocorticoid exposure (>5 mg daily for 3 months or more)
History of hip fracture in parents
Diagnosis of rheumatoid arthritis
Diagnosis of secondary osteoporosis

○ Peripheral sites of DEXA scanning (i.e. wrist) are less sensitive than central sites (hip, spine); **if suspicion is high, a normal study at the wrist should prompt testing of central sites for osteoporosis**

○ Low bone mineral density (BMD) is not always primary osteoporosis and may indicate another medical condition, see Causes of secondary osteoporosis

○ Spine measurements may be falsely elevated or normal in patients with significant osteophytes or aortic calcification at the site of measurement

- Fracture Risk Assessment Tool (FRAX)

  ○ Developed because DEXA scanning in clinical practice has proven specific, but not sensitive, for identification of patients at high risk of fracture – retrospective studies showed that up to 50% of women with postmenopausal fragility fractures **did not** have osteoporosis by DEXA scan

  ○ FRAX incorporates **clinical risk factors** (Table 10.2) to predict the 10-year risk of hip or other major osteoporotic fracture in an individual patient

  ○ The National Osteoporosis Foundation (NOF) FRAX tool is available for clinician use at www.shef.ac.uk/FRAX

**Causes of secondary osteoporosis**

Diabetes
Osteogenesis imperfecta
Hyperthyroidism
Hypogonadism
Early menopause
GI causes: chronic malabsorption or chronic liver disease

- ○ Limitations of FRAX assessment:
  - Does not include bone turnover markers due to lack of data, although the authors propose this may be included in the future
  - Does not include DEXA measured at peripheral sites (but peripheral site measurements lack sensitivity anyway)
  - Study population is still mostly women, limiting generalizability
- Who should be screened for osteoporosis?
  - ○ All females aged >65 years, males >70 years
  - ○ Postmenopausal women and men aged >50 years based on risk factor profile
  - ○ Anyone with an insufficiency fracture, to determine severity of disease
  - ○ Females on hormone replacement therapy
  - ○ Patients on glucocorticoid therapy of >7.5 mg/day for longer than 3 months
- Who should be treated for osteoporosis? National Osteoporosis Foundation (NOF) guidelines
  - ○ Any patient who has suffered an insufficiency fracture
  - ○ Osteoporosis defined by BMD T score ≤ −2.5
  - ○ Postmenopausal women and men aged >50 with T score between −1 and −2.5 with a FRAX score showing 10-year hip fracture risk >3% or 10-year major osteoporotic fracture risk >20%

**Keep in mind**

FRAX treatment thresholds are country specific and are determined by cost effectiveness at each location.

- Markers of bone resorption: a biomarker for osteoporosis?
  - NTx, CTx are **collagen X-linked telopeptides** of type I collagen that are released during osteoclast activity and subsequent collagen breakdown
  - Elevated levels >50 ng/mL may suggest faster bone turnover and increased fracture risk
  - Lower levels after initiation of osteoporosis treatment may suggest treatment response or be used to judge treatment adherence
  - Limitations:
    - Marked physiologic variability and diurnal variability makes a single value difficult to interpret
    - Clinical relevance not well established

## Therapeutic options

- Basic interventions – Institute of Medicine (IOM) recommendations
  - Calcium >1200 mg/day – calcium carbonate is the most cost effective, while calcium citrate may be used if GI upset is an issue
  - Vitamin D >800 mg/day
  - Check total body vitamin D stores, prescribe ergocalciferol if vitamin D <20 ng/mL
  - Weight-bearing exercise
  - Tobacco cessation
  - Limit alcohol and caffeine consumption
  - Once a pharmacologic agent has been started, repeat DEXA should be performed to monitor response every 2 years

---

### Keep in mind

Recommendations for regular calcium and vitamin D supplementation apply only to patients **with** osteoporosis. For patients **without** osteoporosis, new data suggest that calcium and vitamin D supplementation as primary prevention against osteoporosis does not decrease the incidence of fractures, and may increase the risk of heart disease. Therefore, the US Preventive Services Task Force now recommends against routine supplementation of calcium and vitamin D in healthy patients without osteoporosis or other chronic diseases.

**Table 10.3** Regulators of bone remodeling.

| Cell type | Cell origin and function |
| --- | --- |
| Osteoclasts | Derived from hematopoietic stem cells<br>Induce bone resorption |
| Osteoblasts | Derived from local mesenchymal cells<br>Deposits osteoid to promote bone formation<br>Paracrine regulation of osteoclasts |
| Osteocytes | Derived from osteoblasts buried into deposited bone matrix<br>Secrete cytokines, prostaglandins in response to<br>mechanical loading to influence new bone formation |

- **Bisphosphonates** – antiresorptive
  - Alendronate
  - Risedronate
  - Ibandronate
  - Zoledronic acid
  - Mechanism of action
    - Inhibition of osteoclast function (Table 10.3)
    - Promotion of osteoclast apoptosis
    - Tight binding to hydroxyapatite crystal matrix means bisphosphonates will remain active in bone for years; it is continuously released and rebound during cycle of bone remodeling
  - Limitations
    - PO forms cause GI upset and have poor absorption unless taken on an empty stomach
    - IV form can cause infusion reactions, myalgias, and transient flu-like syndrome
    - Osteonecrosis of the jaw (ONJ)
    - Atypical femoral neck fractures

### Keep in mind

All bisphosphonates have been shown to decrease the incidence of vertebral fractures, but only **alendronate** and **risedronate** have been shown to decrease the incidence of hip and non-vertebral osteoporotic fractures.

## Severe adverse events associated with bisphosphonates

### Osteonecrosis of the jaw (ONJ)

ONJ was increasingly reported in case reports and case series beginning in 2006 as an adverse event related to IV and PO bisphosphonate use. This was primarily in the oncology literature due to the regular use of zoledronic acid in patients with painful bony metastases from myeloma, prostate, and breast cancer. ONJ presents as severe pain in the mandible or maxilla, with associated exposed bone and sinus tracts. Pathologic fractures may occur. The majority of cases occur in women, after oral surgery or instrumentation. The highest risk appears to be in patients receiving monthly zoledronic acid or pamidronate for malignancy. Although the exact cause is unknown, it is theorized that bisphosphonate suppression of bone turnover and angiogenesis induces microtrauma and subsequent microfracture, which then leads to localized osteonecrosis. The presence of caries or periodontal disease does appear to play a role. The frequency of ONJ in cancer-free patients receiving bisphosphonates for osteoporosis is unknown, but much less common, with fewer than 20 cases reported in the literature. Treatment is largely preventive, with the American Academy of Oral Medicine recommending a dental exam and any oral surgery required be performed prior to initiation of bisphosphonates, especially if used for cancer treatment. Dental instrumentation should be avoided in patients on bisphosphonate therapy; preliminary data is mixed regarding use of NTx and CTx to predict higher risk of ONJ. Once ONJ develops, treatment is supportive. Bisphosphonates should be discontinued, and antibiotic rinses may be used to promote healing.

### Atypical femoral fractures

Beginning in 2005, several cases of subtrochanteric femoral fractures were reported in patients on alendronate for 5–10 years. These patients exhibited a unique x-ray pattern and typically the fractures occurred without trauma. It is hypothesized that bisphosphonate impairment of normal bone remodeling caused microfractures that increased bone fragility in atypical areas. Atypical fractures were noted more often in patients on glucocorticoid therapy. Two registries examined the link in 2009. The first noted that the incidence of atypical femoral fractures and typical fractures was similar in both bisphosphonate-treated and bisphosphonate-naïve patients. The second noted that atypical fractures occurred at a rate of 1 per 1000/year in bisphosphonate-treated patients, but that this risk is significantly lower than the risk of an osteoporotic hip fracture if not on bisphosphonate therapy. Given the limited data, the FDA concluded there was no definitive evidence of long-term bisphosphonate use and atypical fracture. However, it was noted that there may be diminished benefit to improvement in BMD beyond 5 years of therapy with bisphosphonates. This has led to clinicians considering "drug holidays" after 5 continuous years of bisphosphonate therapy, and the use of the FRAX tool to identify patients who are at low risk of osteoporotic fracture and whose potential benefit from bisphosphonate use may not exceed the possible risk of atypical femoral fracture.

- **Teriperatide** – anabolic
  - Recombinant human parathyroid hormone approved for use in 2002
  - Administered in daily subcutaneous injection for intermittent rPTH exposure
    - **Continuous** PTH exposure increases osteoclast activity and bone loss, however. . .
    - **Intermittent** PTH exposure stimulates bone formation
  - Decreases incidence of vertebral and osteoporotic hip and non-vertebral fractures
  - The only available **anabolic** agent – i.e. actively stimulates bone formation instead of preventing further bone loss
  - A double-blind, placebo-controlled trial of over 1500 patients with osteoporosis and history of vertebral fracture showed teriperatide to decrease the risk of subsequent vertebral fracture by 65%, and risk of subsequent non-vertebral fracture by 53%
  - Limitations
    - Treatment course limited to 2 years due to limited safety/efficacy data after 2 years
    - Increases the risk of osteosarcoma and other malignant bone tumors
    - Should not be used concomitantly with bisphosphonates; patients taking both teriperatide and a bisphosphonate had **reduced** lumbar spine BMD at end of study
    - Therefore these drugs are given in series, with bisphosphonates to start after 1–2 years of teriperatide
- **Denosumab** – antiresorptive
  - Approved in 2010 for first-line treatment of osteoporosis in post-menopausal women

○ Humanized monoclonal antibody directed against RANKL – functions as an OPG analog

○ Given as a subcutaneous injection every 6 months

○ This is the first antiresorptive agent approved for use in patients with renal insufficiency or on dialysis

○ Inhibits osteoclast proliferation and function

○ FREEDOM Trial

- Over 6000 women randomized to placebo or denosumab

- Primary endpoint: new vertebral fracture at 36 months

- Secondary endpoint: time to first non-vertebral fracture or hip fracture

- Denosumab-treated patients had 68% reduction in new vertebral fractures, as well as significant reduction in hip and non-vertebral fractures

- BMD improved in denosumab group

○ Limitations

- No difference in major adverse events (serious infection, malignancy, ONJ, hypercalcemia)

- Denosumab-treated group had more eczema, flatulence, skin infections

- FREEDOM Trial excluded patients with severe osteoporosis due to ethical concerns over placing this population on placebo, therefore there are no data on the efficacy of denosumab in this population

## Further reading

Body, J.J., Gaich, G.A., Scheele, W.H., et al. (2002) A randomized double-blind trial to compare the efficacy of teriparatide with alendronate in postmenopausal women with osteoporosis. *Journal of Clinical Endocrinology & Metabolism* 87(10): 4528–4535.

Cummings, S.R., Martin, J.S., McClung, M.R., et al. (2009) Denosumab for prevention of fractures in postmenopausal women with osteoporosis. *New England Journal of Medicine* 361(8): 756–765.

Kanis, J.A., McCloskey, E.V., Johansson, H., et al. (2010) Development and use of FRAX in osteoporosis. *Osteoporosis International* 21(Suppl 2): S407–413.

Lindsay, R., Nieves, J., Formica, C., et al. (1997) Randomised controlled study of effect of parathyroid hormone on vertebral bone mass and fracture incidence among postmenopausal women on estrogen with osteoporosis. *Lancet* 350(9077): 550–555.

National Osteoporosis Foundation (2008) *Clinician's Guide to Prevention and Treatment of Osteoporosis*. Washington, DC: National Osteoporosis Foundation.

Neer, R.M., Arnaud, C.D., Zanchetta, J.R., et al. (2001) Effect of parathyroid hormone (1–34) on fractures and bone mineral density in postmenopausal women with osteoporosis. *New England Journal of Medicine* 344(19): 1434–1441.

CHAPTER 11

# Review of musculoskeletal radiology

## John Payan, Gnanesh Patel, Karen Law

Emory University School of Medicine, Atlanta, GA, USA

## Introduction

Imaging in the rheumatic diseases is often a key component of diagnosis and management. This section will review classic radiographic features of rheumatoid arthritis, psoriatic arthritis, crystalline arthropathies, and other syndromes commonly seen in the field of rheumatology.

## Radiographic features of RA

- Symmetric and polyarticular joint involvement
- Predilection for hands (MCP, PIP), wrists, and feet (MTP), but elbows, knees, shoulders, and hips also can be affected in aggressive or longstanding disease
- Cervical spine involvement also occurs including facet erosions, cranial settling, and C1–C2 subluxation
- Early manifestations (Figure 11.1)
  - Periarticular soft tissue swelling
  - Periarticular osteopenia
  - Marginal erosions – begin at "bare areas" – intercapsular articular margins, usually at the **ulnar styloid**, **MCP 2 and 3**, and the **fifth MTP** before other areas are affected
- Late manifestations (Figures 11.2, 11.3)
  - Diffuse osteopenia
  - Joint space narrowing

*Rheumatology Board Review*, First Edition. Edited by Karen Law and Aliza Lipson.
© 2014 John Wiley & Sons, Inc. Published 2014 by John Wiley & Sons, Inc.

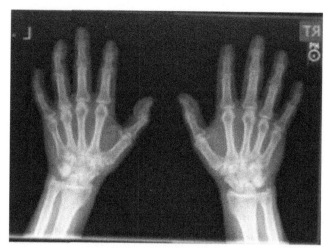

**Figure 11.1** Early rheumatoid arthritis. Primarily periarticular osteopenia; diffuse joint space narrowing; early marginal erosive changes most evident at right second and third and left fourth and fifth MCP and carpal bones

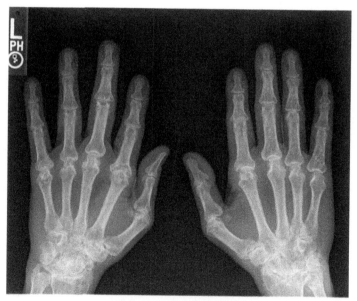

**Figure 11.2** Advanced RA. Diffuse osteopenia; marked joint space narrowing; erosive changes at PIPs, MCPs, radiocarpal, and intercarpal joints at both proximal and distal phalanges.

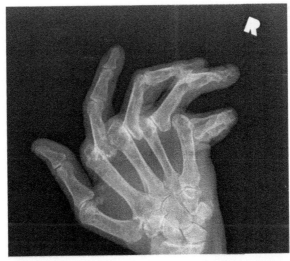

**Figure 11.3** Rheumatoid arthritis with chronic deformities. Diffuse osteopenia; subluxation and ulnar dislocation of the second through fifth MCP joints as sequelae of erosive disease.

- Erosions at both proximal and distal phalanges
- Ulnar deviation
- Joint subluxation and dislocation with characteristic deformities
  - Swan-neck deformity – hyperextension at PIP and flexion at DIP
  - Boutonniere deformity – flexion at PIP and hyperextension at DIP
  - Windswept deformity – symmetric ulnar subluxations and dislocations of the MCP and PIP joints
  - Hitchhiker's thumb: flexion of MCP and hyperextension at IP joint

**Keep in mind**

Windswept deformity can occur in SLE and Jaccoud's arthropathy as well, but typically in the absence of erosive changes customarily seen in RA.

- Ankylosis (fusion) of joints – most often carpals and tarsals
- Secondary osteoarthritic changes: osteophyte formation, subchondral sclerosis, subchondral cyst
See Figures 11.4, 11.5.

**Keep in mind**

**Bilateral protrusio acetabuli deformity** can occur in the following:
- Rheumatoid arthritis
- Ankylosing spondylitis
- Paget's disease
- Marfan's syndrome
- Osteomalacia
- Metastatic disease

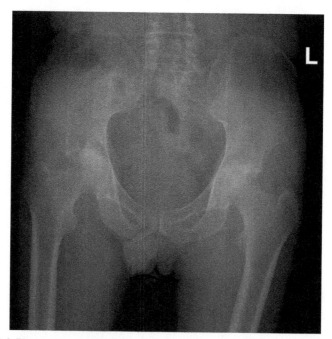

**Figure 11.4** Rheumatoid arthritis affecting the hips. Continued marked diffuse osteopenia; concentric decrease in hip joint space and symmetric cartilage loss; axial migration of the femoral head with resultant acetabular remodeling resulting in protrusio acetabuli deformity; femoral head shows small erosions.

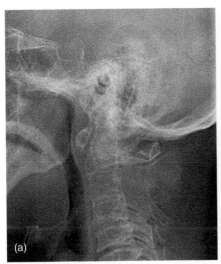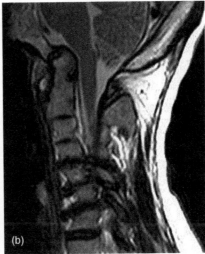

**Figure 11.5 (a,b)** Cervical spine complications of RA: Cranial settling. Inflammation due to RA in the cervical spine causes synovial thickening around the odontoid process of C2. When untreated, this progresses into an inflamed, granulated sheet of tissue called a **rheumatoid pannus** that invades into subchondral bone. The rheumatoid pannus induces bony erosion and destruction of the C1/C2 facets and the stabilizing articulations. As a result, the skull "settles" on to the spinal column and the odontoid migrates superiorly into the foramen magnum, leading to compression of the spinal cord and brainstem between the odontoid and the skull, visible on MRI (**b**). Cranial settling is a neurosurgical emergency, and can lead to neurologic defects, respiratory depression, and sudden death; any complaints of neck pain in a patient with RA require urgent evaluation with plain films, and a low threshold for proceeding with CT/MRI for further evaluation.

# Radiographic features of psoriatic arthritis

**Keep in mind**

There are five patterns of psoriatic arthritis:
- "Classic" form primarily involving the distal joints of hands and feet
- Symmetric arthritis that mimics RA (but is RF negative)
- Asymmetric arthritis with sausage digits
- Spondylitis with peripheral arthritis
- Arthritis mutilans – a severe, deforming, and destructive arthritis that can occur in RA as well

- Polyarticular inflammatory arthritis affecting primarily the joints of the hands and feet
- Bone density is normal
- DIP involvement is common; wrist involvement is rare
- Joint involvement is typically asymmetric
- Early erosive changes progress to severe subchondral erosions, primarily at proximal phalanges of involved joints (Figure 11.6)
- Enthesophytes can be seen at sites of enthesopathy (Figure 11.7)
- Soft tissue swelling may involve the entire digit, termed a "sausage digit" or dactylitis
- Productive change or periostitis occurs at distal articular surfaces of involved joints as well as along the length of involved phalanges
- Advanced disease can produce a classic "pencil in cup" deformity with erosion of the proximal phalanx into a "pencil," and productive changes along the distal periarticular surface into a "cup" (Figure 11.8)
- Arthropathy may precede the development of psoriasis in up to 20% of patients
- Figure 11.9 illustrates telescoping digits and arthritis mutilans. See also Table 11.1

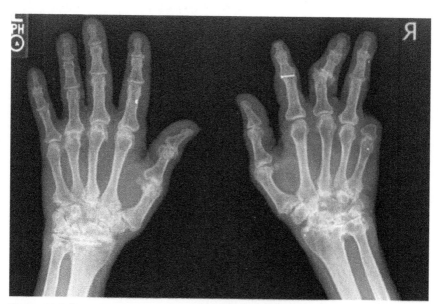

**Figure 11.6** Psoriatic arthritis in the hands. Asymmetric joint involvement; erosive changes in left MCP 2, 3, 4; erosive and proliferative changes in right PIP 3; milder DIP involvement evident in left DIP 2 and right DIP 2 and 3; mild soft tissue swelling of entire left second digit consistent with dactylitis.

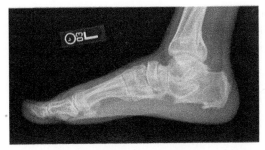

**Figure 11.7** Enthesophytes at sites of enthesopathy. Plantar calcaneal enthesophyte.

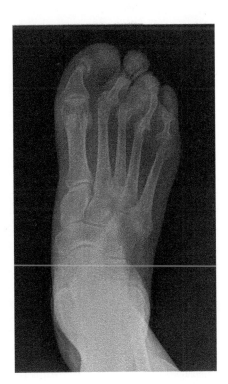

**Figure 11.8** Psoriatic arthritis in the foot. Note complete erosion of the articular surface at MTP 3; great toe with early pencil in cup deformity at the IP joint: destruction and resorption of the middle phalanx with bony proliferation at the distal phalangeal base; generalized soft tissue swelling consistent with dactylitis.

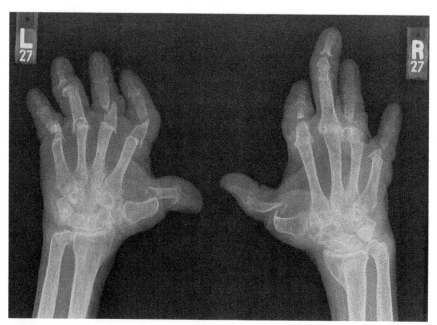

**Figure 11.9** Telescoping digits. Marked bone erosion and resorption has obliterated the articular surfaces, resulting in complete loss of left PIPs 2–5 and right PIPs 2, 4, 5; clinically this manifests as telescoping digits and arthritis mutilans from psoriatic arthritis.

**Table 11.1** Distinguishing psoriatic arthritis from rheumatoid arthritis.

|  | Psoriatic arthritis | Rheumatoid arthritis |
|---|---|---|
| Symmetric joint involvement | No | Yes |
| Juxta-articular osteopenia | No | Yes |
| DIP involvement | Yes | No |
| Wrist involvement | Rare | Common |
| Dactylitis | Yes | No |
| Periostitis | Yes | No |
| Enthesophytes | Yes | No |
| Subchondral cysts | Rare | Common |

# Radiographic features of ankylosing spondylitis

- Mixed erosive and productive arthritis
- Involves primarily the axial skeleton and may involve the large proximal joints

- Sacroiliac joint involvement is a hallmark of the disease, more prominently on the inferior, iliac side of the joint (the synovial portion) in early disease but later involving the entire joint

---

**Keep in mind**

Sacroiliitis in AS is typically **bilateral** and **symmetric**. **Unilateral** or **asymmetric sacroiliitis** is more consistent with RA, psoriatic arthritis, or reactive arthritis.

---

- The superior pole of the sacroiliac joint is made primarily of ligaments that can form **bridging enthesophytes**
- Bridging enthesophytes can also be seen in:
  - DISH
  - Chronic reactive arthritis
  - Psoriatic arthritis
  - Vitamin D toxicity
- Disease progression leads to sacroiliac joint fusion and subsequent progression cranially to involve the thoracolumbar spine
- Vertebral involvement begins at the peripheral corners of the vertebral body, where enthesitis and reactive sclerosis induces the **"shiny corner" sign**
- Subsequent erosion at the peripheral corners of vertebral bodies induces loss of normal concavity, leading to a squared appearance of vertebral bodies on lateral films (Figure 11.10)
- Further progression of the disease in the thoracolumbar spine includes ossificiation of the annulus fibrosis, or syndesmophytes
- End stages of ankylosing spondylitis show ankylosis or fusion of the vertebral bodies into the classic finding of **"bamboo spine"** (Figure 11.11)

---

**Keep in mind**

Basilar invagination (BI) and atlantoaxial subluxation (AAS) (Figures 11.12, 11.13) can be seen in RA and AS. These are neurosurgical emergencies, therefore any complaints of neck pain in patients with AS or RA must be further investigated.

---

- Figure 11.14 illustrates the complications of ankylosing spondylitis

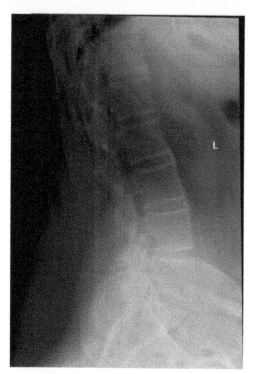

**Figure 11.10** Early vertebral involvement. Lateral film shows squaring of the vertebral bodies; later finding of irregular new bone formation is evident at the corners of some more inferior vertebral bodies. Two vertical syndesmophytes are also evident.

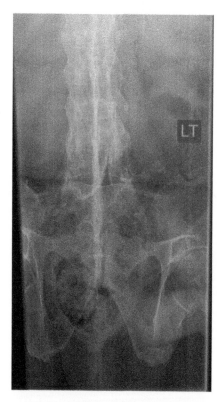

**Figure 11.11** Advanced ankylosing spondylitis: Sacroilitis and bamboo spine. Complete SI joint fusion and advanced AS; fusion of the lumbar vertebral bodies; vertical syndesmophytes are continuous throughout the lumbar spine, giving the characteristic **bamboo spine** appearance; fusion of the intraspinous ligament is also evident, known as the **"dagger sign"**.

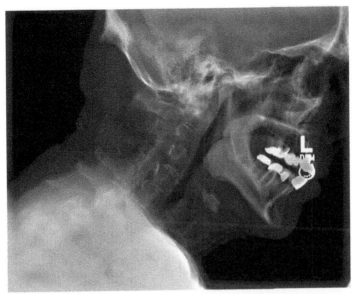

**Figure 11.12** Cervical spine manifestations of AS. C1 vertebral body erosion causing cranial settling and loss of axial supporting structures; the superior portion of C2 (dens) migrates upward to breach the foramen magnum, resulting in **basilar invagination** (BI) and placing the patient at risk for lower brainstem compression or atlantoaxial subluxation (AAS) and cord compression; fusion of the posterior laminae and mild squaring of the vertebral bodies are also evident.

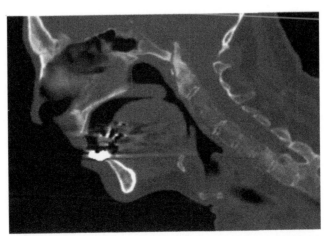

**Figure 11.13** Sagittal view of AS in the cervical spine. CT sagittal reconstruction showing protrusion of the dens upward into the foramen magnum, causing brainstem compression.

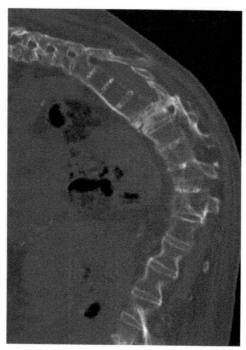

**Figure 11.14** Complications of ankylosing spondylitis. One of the most serious complications of AS is spinal fracture after minor trauma, seen here in this CT sagittal spine; spinal fracture at the midthoracic spine is evident, due to kyphosis, diffuse osteopenia, and rigidity from ankylosis. Spinal fracture at either the cervicothoracic or thoracolumbar junction is most common due to instability at these primary flexion points in the spine. Therefore, any AS patient presenting with new pain, especially at primary flexion points, must be evaluated for fracture or pseudoarthrosis that may result in paralysis.

## Radiographic findings in crystalline arthropathies

### Gout

- Asymmetric and monoarticular or polyarticular arthritis
- Radiographic findings are generally not visible for many years, typically 7–10 years after initial clinical and laboratory manifestations
- Feet are most commonly involved; primarily the first MTP, but also other MTPs, IP joints, and tarsal bones
- In the hands, DIP, PIP, MCP, and intercarpal joints can be affected; olecranon erosions and olecranon tophi in the bursa can also occur
- Erosions in gout are typically well defined, with sclerotic margins leading to a "punched out" appearance on plain films
- Overhanging edges are also evident from new bone formation (Figure 11.15)

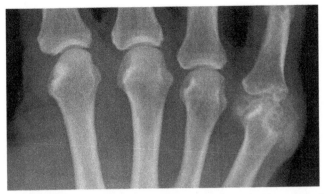

**Figure 11.15** Erosive gout. Erosion at the fifth metacarpal head with overhanging edges; overlying soft tissue swelling; relative preservation of the joint space; soft tissue calcification of the tophus; bone density is maintained.

- Normal or near-normal bone density
- Joint spaces are well preserved until late in the disease, helping to differentiate from other erosive arthropathies
- Calcification of tophi can occur, usually with a "cloud-like" pattern (Figure 11.16)
- Gout can coexist with CPPD or infection
- Can lead to non-traumatic tendon rupture (which can also occur in RA, SLE, diabetes, obesity, fluoroquinolone use)
- Figure 11.17 shows advanced tophaceous gout

## Calcium pyrophosphate disease
- Typical finding is chondrocalcinosis, or calcium deposition in cartilage, synovium, or joint capsule
- Typical sites of involvement include the menisci of the knees (Figure 11.18), triangular fibrocartilage (TFC) of the wrist (Figure 11.19), proximal joints of the hand, pubic symphysis, acetabular labrum, and annular ligament of the spine
- Can be seen in association with hemochromatosis; the presence of **hook osteophytes** and osteoarthritis of MCPs 2 and 3 with chondrocalcinosis can raise the suspicion for concomitant hemochromatosis (Figure 11.20)
- The disease exhibits primarily productive changes with osteophytes and sclerosis, though erosive changes may occur
- Although radiographic appearance may mimic osteoarthritis, the location of abnormalities and symmetric distribution in CPPD helps to distinguish the two
- Bone density is usually normal
- May have large subchondral cysts

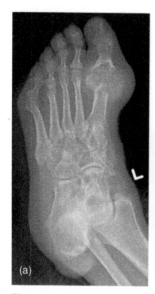
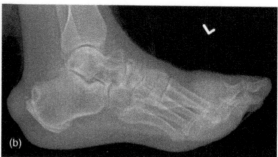

**Figure 11.16 (a,b)** Longstanding gout in the foot. Destruction of the first MTP and proximal aspect of the proximal phalanx of the great toe is seen; cloud-like calcification and tophi around the first MTP and posterior aspect of the calcaneus are evident; punched out erosions of the dorsal aspect of the talar and navicular bones and a large bony erosion at the posterior aspect of the calcaneus are evident.

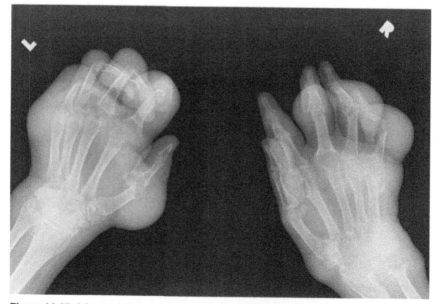

**Figure 11.17** Advanced tophaceous gout. Advanced tophaceous arthritis with near total osteolysis of most of the right carpal bones and heavy tophus burden, especially over PIPs.

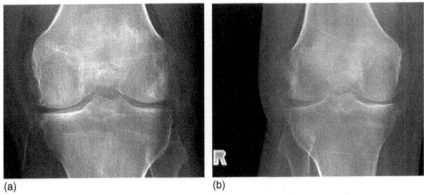

(a)                                    (b)

**Figures 11.18 (a,b)** Bilateral knee CPPD. Chondrocalcinosis seen as a linear density within menisci of knees bilaterally; note bilateral bony erosions of the lateral femoral condyles that may mimic gout, but represent CPPD in this bilateral, symmetric distribution and clinical setting. **Osteoarthritis of the patellofemoral joint is more common in CPPD versus the typical medial joint compartment in conventional OA, typically detectable in a lateral film.**

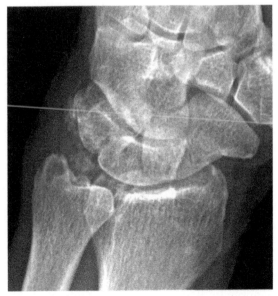

**Figure 11.19** Chondrocalcinosis in the wrist. TFC chondrocalcinosis; large subchondral cystic changes in the ulnar styloid.

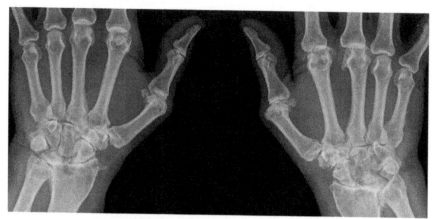

**Figure 11.20** Advanced CPPD of the hand. Multiple cystic lucencies throughout the carpal bones, distal radius, and distal ulna bilaterally; complete loss of the normal radiocarpal joint space. **SLAC wrist** is a typical deformity from CPPD due to proximal migration of the capitate between the dissociated scaphoid and lunate bone. Also evident is loss of joint space at the right second and third MCP joints with large **hook-like osteophytes** and subchondral cyst formation which can suggest hemochromatosis.

---

**Keep in mind**

SLAC wrist may also occur in RA, post-traumatic damage, and in CPPD.

---

## Radiographic features of diffuse idiopathic skeletal hyperostosis (DISH)

- An idiopathic disease that causes ossification of the soft tissues of the spine, including the paravertebral connective tissues, annulus fibrosis, and anterior longitudinal ligament, over four contiguous levels (Figure 11.21)
- Typically involves the thoracic spine most commonly, followed by cervical and lumbar spine involvement
- Ossification of the anterior longitudinal ligament results in thick, bulky, flowing syndesmophytes that can be confused with those seen in ankylosing spondylitis (Figure 11.22, Table 11.2)
- Sacroiliac joint involvement may be seen, in which the superior (ligamentous) pole of the sacroiliac joint exhibits ossification and fusion, while the inferior (synovial) pole is typically normal

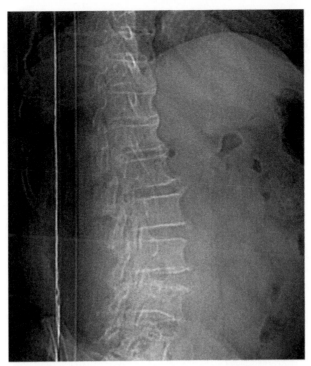

**Figure 11.21** Early DISH in the lower thoracic spine. Early development of ossification of the anterior longitudinal ligament along the anterolateral aspect of the spine over four levels. Unlike in AS, ossification in DISH is not continuous and is not associated with loss of disc height or squaring of the vertebral bodies.

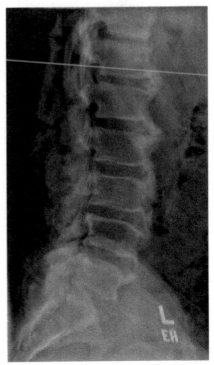

**Figure 11.22** DISH in the lumbar spine. Dense, **bulky** ossification of the anterior longitudinal ligament over four contiguous segments. Note continued preserved disc height and lack of squaring of vertebral bodies.

> ### Keep in mind
>
> Sacroiliac joint inflammation in AS, in contrast to DISH, typically begins at the **inferior pole of the SI joint**.

- Figure 11.23 illustrates DISH in the cervical spine

**Table 11.2** Differentiating ankylosing spondylitis and DISH.

|  | AS | DISH |
|---|---|---|
| SI joint involvement | Primarily inferior (synovial) portion | Primarily superior (ligamentous) portion |
| Continuous spine involvement without skip areas | Yes | No |
| ALL ossification | Thin, delicate | Thick, bulky |
| Shiny corner sign | Yes | No |
| Squaring of vertebral bodies | Yes | No |

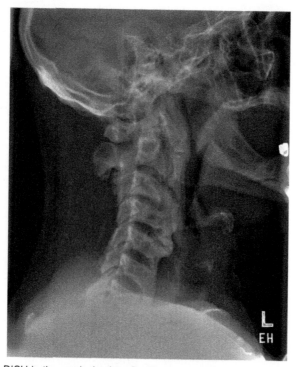

**Figure 11.23** DISH in the cervical spine. Ossification of both the anterior and posterior longitudinal ligaments, which can be seen in up to 50% of patients with DISH. Bulky ossification may cause significant esophageal impingement during swallowing, if anterior, or cervical spinal cord compression, if posterior.

# Radiographic features of sarcoidosis

- Systemic granulomatous disease that affects the lung and other internal organs in addition to the joints (Figures 11.24, 11.25)
- About 10% of patients with sarcoidosis exhibit bone or joint involvement
- Bone or joint involvement with sarcoidosis in the absence of chest x-ray findings consistent with sarcoidosis is **exceedingly rare**
- Typical joint and bone involvement shows "lacy," reticular lytic lesions in the middle or distal phalanges of the fingers
  - These areas represent areas of granulomatous infiltration of the medullary cavity of the bone
- Sclerosis of articular surfaces may also occur
- Pathologic fractures at sites of lesions are common

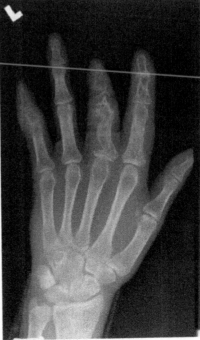

**Figure 11.24** Sarcoidosis in the hand. Typical **lacy lytic lesions** in the middle and distal phalanges, most notably in the second, third, and fifth digits. Accompanying soft tissue swelling can mimic dactylitis and in these cases spondyloarthropathy must also be on the differential diagnosis list. There is a pathologic fracture of the third digit due to granulomatous infiltration.

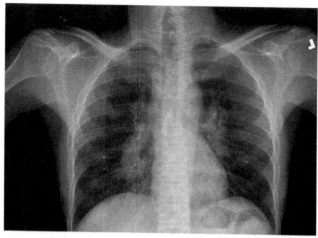

**Figure 11.25** Same patient, chest x-ray. Classic pattern of sarcoidosis in the lung, with pronounced bilateral hilar and right paratracheal lymphadenopathy and pulmonary infiltrates.

# Radiographic features of septic and neuropathic arthropathy

## Septic arthropathy
- Suspicion should be high in the typical clinical settings of fever, soft tissue swelling, overlying skin trauma, and monoarticular involvement
- Initial radiographs of septic arthritis may only show effusion and soft tissue swelling, with hazy articular surfaces
- More chronic infections will show joint space narrowing, periarticular osteoporosis, and adjacent bone, cartilage, and soft tissue destruction with sclerotic margins (Figure 11.26)
- Tuberculous and fungal infections are more indolent and therefore damage may progress more slowly
- Depending on the organism, gas or fluid collections may be present
- Septic arthropathy may be distinguished from gout by the level of surrounding soft tissue destruction and tendency for the arthritis to spread extensively across joint spaces

## Neuropathic arthropathy (Charcot joint)
- Common conditions associated with neuropathic arthropathy include
  - **Diabetes:** associated with Lisfranc injury, in which the tarsal bones are displaced from the tarsus (midfoot) due to repetitive subclinical trauma (Figure 11.27)

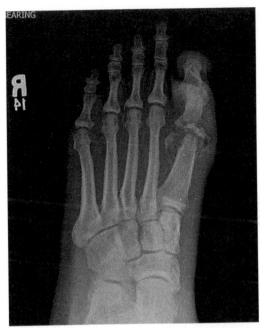

**Figure 11.26** Septic arthropathy of the great toe. Note the extensive inflammation on both sides of the involved joint spaces.

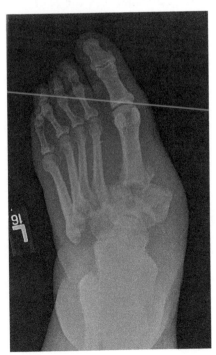

**Figure 11.27** Charcot of the foot. Classic midfoot bony and ligamentous destruction consistent with Lisfranc deformity, a specific form of neuropathic arthropathy. Lisfranc deformity involves ligamentous destruction of the midfoot leading to lateral displacement of digits 2–5; clinically this manifests as lateral deviation of digits 2–5 away from the great toe. Note normal bone density and bony debris in the midfoot.

○ **Syringomyelia**: associated with neuropathic shoulder primarily
○ **Spinal cord injury**: typical joint involved depends on the level of spinal cord injury
○ **Multiple sclerosis**
○ **Chronic alcoholism**: typically involves the foot and/or the knee
○ **Amyloidosis**
○ **Syphilis**: typically involves the knee

• Joint destruction results from chronic microtrauma and altered innervation of local bone and soft tissue, leading to abnormal healing and a cycle of chronic injury
• Joint instability and large effusions are common, with marked associated soft tissue swelling and ligamentous injury
• Typical findings are known as the five Ds:
  ○ Normal bone density
  ○ Joint distension
  ○ Bony debris and interarticular bodies
  ○ Joint disorganization
  ○ Dislocation
• Superimposed infection, especially in diabetic patients, may occur, and often septic arthritis and neuropathic arthritis are difficult to distinguish from one another
• In these situations MRI with contrast can demonstrate soft tissue abscess and/or sinus tract indicating osteomyelitis

## Radiographic features of Paget's disease of the bone

• Disrupted osteoclast and osteoblast equilibrium leads to progressive skeletal deformities (Figure 11.28)
• Most common areas of involvement include the pelvis, followed by hips and tibia, lumbar spine and sacrum, skull, and shoulder
• Three phases of disease:
  1. **Osteolytic phase**: osteoclastic bone resorption
  2. **Mixed lytic and blastic phase**: osteoblasts are activated to counteract osteoclast activities
  3. **Sclerotic phase**
• Disorganized bone resorption causes typical radiographic findings of cortical and trabecular bone thickening and bone expansion
• Later lytic and blastic activity causes a classic **"cotton wool"** appearance to the cranial skull

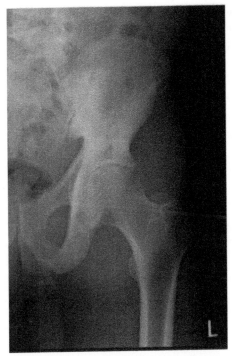

**Figure 11.28** Paget's disease in the left hip. Bone expansion and cortical bone thickening along the femur. **Brim sign** is evident (thickening of the iliopectineal line from body of pubic symphisis towards acetabulum), which is pathognomonic for Paget's disease. There is moderate osteoarthritis of the hip and a **mosaic** appearance to femoral head and adjacent ilium, due to thickened trabecular pattern and bony cortices. The main differential diagnosis with this appearance is blastic metastatic disease due to prostate or breast cancer or lymphoma; as a distinguishing feature, bone tends to be enlarged in Paget's but in malignancy, bony cortical margins are not enlarged.

- Weakened subchondral bone can lead to **early osteoarthritis** and **pathologic fractures**; patients are otherwise typically asymptomatic
- In 1% of cases, Paget's disease can transform into **sarcoma**, usually accompanied by a sudden rise in serum alkaline phosphatase

## Radiographic features of avascular necrosis (AVN)

- Common causes:
  - Steroid use
  - Sickle cell disease
  - Chronic alcoholism
  - HIV

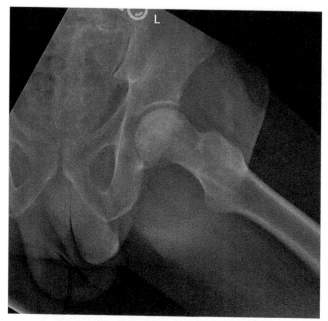

**Figure 11.29** Crescent sign in hip AVN without collapse.

- ○ Idiopathic
- ○ Vasculitis
- ○ Pregnancy
- Classically involves the hips, but may also involve the knees and shoulders
- **Bilateral** hip involvement may be present in 50–80% of cases
- Initial signs of AVN include **sclerosis of the femoral head**; however it may take months for this to be evident on plain film
- MRI is both sensitive and specific at detecting earlier changes
- Over time, a **"crescent sign"** develops – essentially a linear subchondral fracture at the area of sclerosis (Figure 11.29)
- Late findings include **collapse of the femoral head** with secondary osteoarthritis (Figure 11.30)

## Radiographic features of osteoarthritis

- The most common arthropathy
- Cartilage damage results in inadequate cushioning of adjacent subchondral bone and joint space narrowing, resulting in adaptive changes such as osteophyte formation, fibrosis, and sclerosis, as well as joint malalignment and subchondral cyst formation (Figure 11.31)

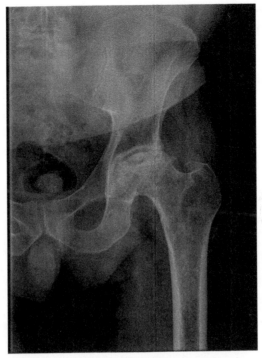

**Figure 11.30** AVN of the hip with collapse of the femoral head and secondary osteoarthritis.

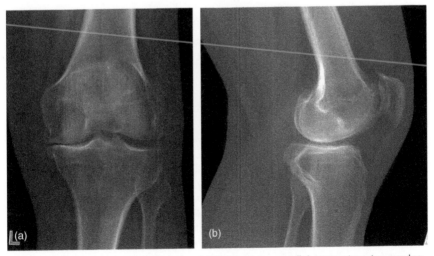

**Figure 11.31** Osteoarthritis of the knee. (**a**) Osteophytes, medial compartment narrowing, and increased height of the tibial spines, consistent with osteoarthritis. (**b**) Subchondral cysts and patellofemoral osteoarthritis. Subchondral sclerosis is also evident at the distal femur and proximal tibia, otherwise there is normal bone density.

- Bone density is normal
- Joint space loss is non-uniform and asymmetric
- Most common locations are the hips, knees, and spine
- Most common locations in the hand are the DIPs, first CMCs, and the scapho-trapezio-trapezoidal complex of the wrist
- Erosive osteoarthritis is a subset of osteoarthritis, most commonly seen in the DIPs and PIPs of the hands in postmenopausal women
- In erosive osteoarthritis, centrally located erosions develop, with more marginal osteophytes, creating a characteristic **"gull wing"** across the articular surface (Figure 11.32)

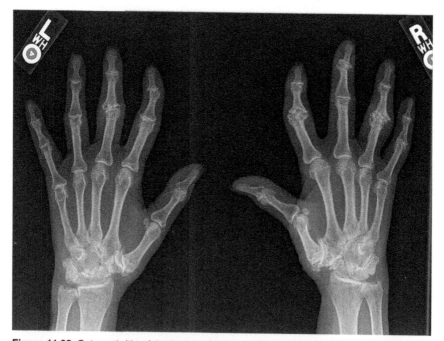

**Figure 11.32** Osteoarthritis of the hands. Symmetric joint involvement is evident with ostearthritic changes notable in DIP, PIP, and first CMC joints of both hands. Proliferative osteophyte changes at the first CMC joints are classic for osteoarthritis, and correlate clinically with "squaring" of the first CMC on physical exam. Subchondral cysts and sclerotic articular margins are evident in the IP joints of both hands, most notably the left second and third PIPs, the right second and fourth PIPs, and the right third DIP. The sclerotic margin in the right second PIP demonstrates the classic **"gull wing" deformity** consistent with erosive osteoarthritis. Note that the bone density throughout the hands is relatively normal.

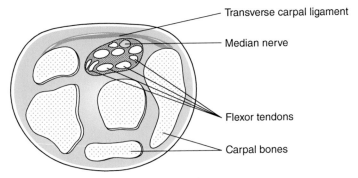

**Color plate 1.1** Components of the carpal tunnel.

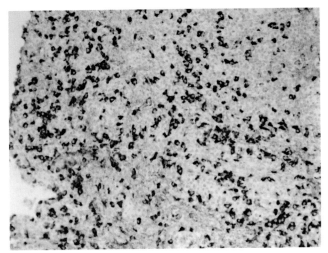

**Color plate 5.1** Immunostaining for IgG4 in IgG4-RD. The majority of plasma cells appear positive for IgG4.

*Rheumatology Board Review*, First Edition. Edited by Karen Law and Aliza Lipson.
© 2014 John Wiley & Sons, Inc. Published 2014 by John Wiley & Sons, Inc.

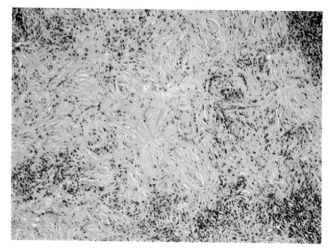

**Color plate 5.2** IgG4-related disease typically shows an irregularly whorled pattern of fibrosis (storiform fibrosis) associated with lymphoplasmacytic infiltration.

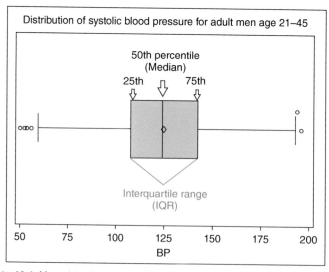

**Color plate 12.1** Mean blood pressure of men.

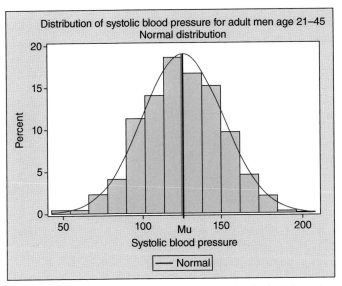

**Color plate 12.2** Normal or Gaussian distribution – example of a bell-shaped curve.

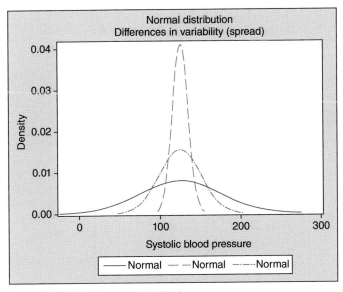

**Color plate 12.3** Variability in normal distribution.

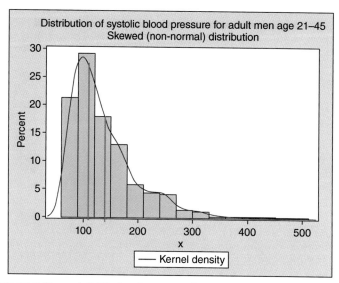

**Color plate 12.4** Skewed distribution (non-normal).

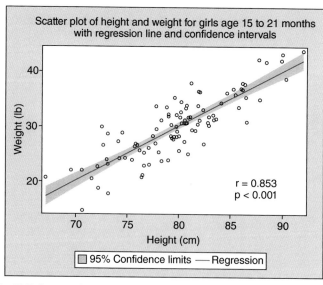

**Color plate 12.5** Scatter plot with best fit line and 95% confidence band (r = Pearson's sample correlation coefficient).

# CHAPTER 12

# Study design, measurement, and basic statistical analysis

## Sheila Angeles-Han, Courtney McCracken

Emory University School of Medicine, Atlanta, GA, USA

## Introduction

Clinical, basic science and translational research studies contribute to an improved understanding of rheumatic diseases and disorders. Ongoing studies can lead to advancement of treatment and better outcomes for our patients. Therefore, a basic knowledge of study design, measurement, and statistical analysis is essential.

## Epidemiologic study designs

Study design is a plan for selecting study subjects and obtaining data about them. Each design is devised to help answer a different type of study question:
- Observational studies
  - **Case control studies**
    - Individuals with disease (cases) are compared to individuals without disease (controls) **retrospectively**
    - Compares frequency of past exposure between cases who develop disease and controls who do not have disease
    - Data determining prior exposure to an agent are obtained
    - The investigator works retrospectively
    - Can calculate odds ratio
  - Cross-sectional
    - A population is observed at one point in time
    - Exposure and outcome are determined at the same point or period in time

*Rheumatology Board Review*, First Edition. Edited by Karen Law and Aliza Lipson.
© 2014 John Wiley & Sons, Inc. Published 2014 by John Wiley & Sons, Inc.

- All measurements are made on a single occasion to determine prevalence of a disease
- Can calculate prevalence
  ○ **Cohort studies**
    - Individuals without disease are monitored prospectively for the development of disease
    - Compares disease incidence over time between groups who have been exposed to a factor of interest
    - Can be retrospective and prospective
- Clinical trials
  ○ Phase 1 – human pharmacology trials to establish initial safety and tolerability of dose range, to assess pharmacodynamics, and to assess drug activity
  ○ Phase 2 – performed to establish efficacy in the intended patient population
  ○ Phase 3 – confirm therapeutic benefit
  ○ Phase 4 – conducted after drug reaches the market to expand on knowledge of the drug's safety, efficacy, and dose

## Common descriptors of data

- Scales of measurement (Table 12.1)
  ○ **Categorical (nominal) variables**
    - Variables that are not quantifiable can be measured by classifying into categories
    - Categories are not ordered
    - Qualitative variables that can be categorized into proportions or percentages
    - Examples: yes and no (dichotomous), blood type, gender
  ○ **Ordinal (ranked) variables**
    - Variables that have an order
    - Although there is order among the categories, the difference between adjacent categories may not be uniform or quantifiable
    - Examples: severity scores of pain (none, mild, moderate, severe)

**Table 12.1** Scales of measurement.

| Scale | Description | Example |
|---|---|---|
| Categorical/nominal | No order | Gender |
| Ordinal/ranked | Ordered, but not quantifiable | Pain scores |
| Continuous/interval | Ordered and quantifiable | Age |

- ○ **Continuous (interval/numerical) variables**
  - ▪ Quantified intervals on an infinite scale of values
  - ▪ Values are ranked
  - ▪ Differences between numbers have meaning on a numerical scale
  - ▪ Examples: age and blood pressure
- • Measures of central tendency – provides data on where data cluster (Figure 12.1)
  - ○ **Mean** – arithmetic average (continuous) or sum of the values divided by the number of values
  - ○ **Median** – centermost value (ranked or ordered categories)
  - ○ **Mode** – most frequently observed value (nominal data)
- • Measures of spread or variation
  - ○ **Standard deviation** – the variability of individual observations or the measure of the spread of the variables (Figure 12.2)
  - ○ **Standard error of the mean** – the variability of means or the range of where the true population mean lies
  - ○ **Confidence interval** – an interval of values within which one is 95% confident that the true population parameter lies. One would expect that 95% of samples drawn from the population would have a sample estimate that fell within the designated confidence limits
- • Bell-shaped curve
  - ○ Normal or Gaussian distribution is a symmetric bell-shaped curve where the mean lies at the central peak, 50% of the distribution lies to

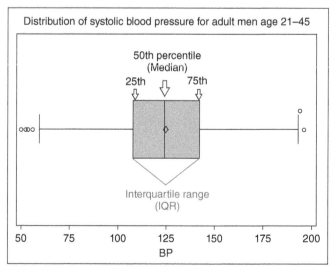

**Figure 12.1** Mean blood pressure of men (Color plate 12.1).

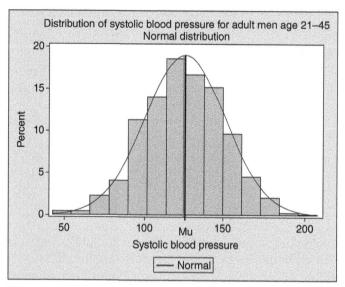

**Figure 12.2** Normal or Gaussian distribution – example of a bell-shaped curve (Color plate 12.2).

the left of the mean, and 50% to the right of the mean (Figures 12.2, 12.3, 12.4)

## Disease frequency and risk factors

- Disease frequency (Table 12.2)
  - **Incidence** – number of new cases over a period of time in a population
    - Incident cases divided by the amount of at-risk population from which they arose
    - $(a+c)/(a+b+c+d)$
  - **Prevalence** – total number of subjects with disease (cases) in a population at risk of developing disease either at a point in time or during a time period
    - These can be given as proportions (0–1), percentages (0–100) or actual cases per population
      - → Number of cases divided by the population at risk
      - → $(a+c)/$size of population $(a+b+c+d)$
    - Point prevalence – number of new and old cases in a population in an instant in time
    - Period prevalence – number of new and old cases in a defined population during a time period

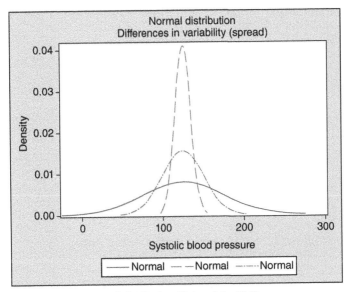

**Figure 12.3** Variability in normal distribution (Color plate 12.3).

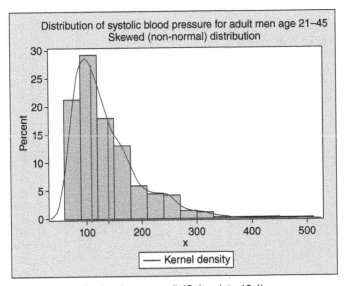

**Figure 12.4** Skewed distribution (non-normal) (Color plate 12.4).

**Table 12.2** Disease frequency and risk factors.

| Risk factor/exposure | Disease present | Disease absent | Total |
|---|---|---|---|
| Present (+) | a | b | a + b |
| Absent (−) | c | d | c + d |
| Total | a + c | b + d | a + b + c + d |

- Risk factors for disease
  - **Risk** – number of new cases in a population at risk
  - **Relative risk** – risk of developing disease in an exposed group compared to risk in an unexposed group
    - Values can range from 0 to infinity
      - → 1 = no difference in risk between the groups
      - → >1 = increased risk
      - → <1 = decreased risk
    - Incidence in those exposed divided by incidence in those not exposed
    (a/[a+b]) / (c/[c+d])
  - **Odds ratio** – approximation of relative risk in retrospective studies
  (a × d)/(b × c)

## Measurement error

See Table 12.3.
- **Sensitivity** – individuals with disease who test positive for disease
  - TP/(TP + FN)
- **Specificity** – individuals without disease who test negative for disease
  - TN/(TN + FP)
- **False positive or type I error** – individuals who test positive but who do not have disease
  - FP/(TP + FP)
- **False negative or type II error** – Individuals who test negative but who do have disease
  - FN/(TN + FN)
- **Positive predictive value** – proportion or percentage of individuals who test positive who do have the disease
  - TP/(TP + FP)
- **Negative predictive value** – proportion or percentage of individuals who test negative who do not have the disease
  - TN/(TN + FN)

**Table 12.3** 2 × 2 table for assessing agreement between test and disease status.

| Test Result | Disease present | Disease absent |
|---|---|---|
| (+) | True positive (TP) | False positive (FP) |
| (−) | False negative (FN) | True negative (TN) |

## Basic statistical tests

- Statistical error and p-values
  - Null hypothesis
    - There is no relationship or association between two variables
    - A study will attempt to reject or disprove the null hypothesis
  - Alternative hypothesis
    - There is a relationship or association between two variables
  - Type I error is the probability of rejecting the null hypothesis when it is true
    - **One concludes there is a significant difference when there is none**
    - Alpha error – level of statistical significance
  - Type II error is the probability of failing to reject the null hypothesis when it is false
    - **One concludes there is not a significant difference where is one**
    - Beta error
  - P-value is the **calculated type I error level** or the **likelihood that a difference at least as large as the observed difference could have occurred by chance alone**
    - Probability of seeing an effect as big or bigger than that in the study by chance if the null hypothesis is true
    - If the calculated p-value is **greater** than the predefined type I error, than the result is **not statistically significant**
    - If the calculated p-value is **at or below** the predefined type I error, than the result **is statistically significant**
- Bivariate relationships or two sample tests (Table 12.4)
  - **Chi-square test**
    - This test is for categorical and ordinal data and is used to assess the **association** between two variables
    - Compares proportion of subjects in two groups who have a dichotomous outcome (two possible values or categories)

○ **Fisher exact test**
  ▪ Replaces the chi-square test when the expected frequency of one or more cells is <5
○ **Student t-test**
  ▪ The student t-test is used for **continuous** data that are **normally distributed** when comparing two groups (Figure 12.2)
  ▪ Determines whether the mean value of a continuous outcome variable in one group differs significantly from another group
  ▪ It can be used for two independent samples
  ▪ For data that are not normally distributed, then non-parametric tests such as the Mann-Whitney U are employed (Figure 12.4)
• Multiple variable relationships (Table 12.4)
  ○ **One-way analysis of variance (ANOVA)**
    ▪ Used to compare **more than two samples or means**
    ▪ Can also use multi-way ANOVA to compare **two or more independent variables on one dependent variable**
    ▪ The Kruskal–Wallis test can be used in samples that are **not normally distributed**

**Table 12.4** Basic statistical tests for comparing two or more groups or finding the association between two continuous measurements.

| Number of groups | Type of outcome measure | Test | Type of test |
|---|---|---|---|
| Two groups | Categorical ordinal/nominal | Chi-square | Non-parametric |
| | Continuous | Student t-test | Parametric |
| | Continuous | Mann–Whitney U (Wilcoxon-Rank Sum) | Non-parametric |
| More than two groups | Categorical ordinal/nominal | Chi-Square | Non-parametric |
| | Continuous | ANOVA | Parametric |
| | Continuous | Kruskal-Wallis test | Non-parametric |
| Association between two continuous variables (no grouping) | Continuous | Pearson's correlation | Parametric |
| | Continuous | Spearman's rho | Non-parametric |
| | Continuous | Linear regression | Parametric |

○ Correlation
  ▪ Coefficients measure the **strength of a linear association** between two variables
  ▪ Magnitude can range between 0.0 to 1.0 using a continuous scale
    → Varies between −1 and +1 wherein negative values indicate as one variable increases, the other decreases
    → There is a stronger association the closer the coefficient is to 1.0 and a weaker association the closer the coefficient is to 0
      ○ Weak correlations – below 0.30
      ○ Moderate correlations – between 0.30 and 0.70
      ○ Strong correlation – above 0.70
  ▪ Pearson's correlation, r, is used for **normally** distributed samples
  ▪ Spearman's rho is the **non-parametric** equivalent of Pearson's correlation
○ Regression
  ▪ A model wherein a predictor or independent variable affects the dependent outcome variable
  ▪ Determines **which independent variables contribute to predictions of the dependent variable**
  ▪ $y = a + bx$
    → a is the intercept; b is the beta coefficient or slope (Figure 12.5)

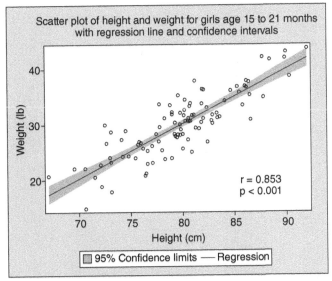

**Figure 12.5** Scatter plot with best fit line and 95% confidence band (r = Pearson's sample correlation coefficient) (Color plate 12.5).

- Multiple regression
  - → Multiple linear regression is when **many independent variables** are investigated **simultaneously** on a continuous dependent variable
    - ○ Can assess the **un-confounded effects** of independent variables
  - → Multiple logistic regression involves regressing independent predictors on a dichotomous response (dependent variable)
    - ○ It is often used to determine **which predictor variables best predict an outcome** (disease vs. no disease)
    - ○ The independent variables can be categorical, ordinal, and continuous
- Survival analysis
  - ○ Determines the amount of time a cohort of subjects **survives**
  - ○ Can compare effective of two treatments in prolonging life or decreasing disease symptoms
  - ○ Fixed-interval (actuarial)
  - ○ Kaplan–Meier survival analysis

## Further reading

Hulley, S.B. (2001) *Designing Clinical Research: an Epidemiologic Approach*, 2nd ed. Philadelphia: Lippincott Williams & Wilkins; xv, 336.

Koepsell, T.D., Weiss, N.S. (2003) *Epidemiologic Methods: Studying the Occurrence of Illness*. Oxford, New York: Oxford University Press; ix, 513.

Nardi, P.M. (2006) *Doing Survey Research: a Guide to Quantitative Methods*, 2nd edn. Boston: Pearson/Allyn & Bacon; xiii, 240.

# CHAPTER 13

# Update on vasculitis

## Karen Law

Emory University School of Medicine, Atlanta, GA, USA

## Introduction

The vasculitides are a heterogeneous set of diseases identified by the presence of blood vessel wall inflammation, with associated tissue and organ damage specific to each disease. Several classification schemas exist; in general the vasculitides are classified based on the size and type of blood vessels affected, as well as the presence or absence of immune deposits and ANCA (Figure 13.1). While, classically, many vasculitides have been known by their eponyms, recent consensus groups recommend a shift towards disease-specific nomenclature. This includes the identification of Churg–Strauss vasculitis as eosinophilc granulomatous polyangiitis (EGPA) and Wegener's granulomatosis as granulomatous polyangiitis (GPA). This chapter will focus on recent updates to the ANCA-associated vasculitides (AAV).

## ANCA-associated vasculitides

The ANCA-associated vasculitides include the following:
- **Granulomatosis with polyangiitis** (GPA, previously Wegener's granulomatosis)
- **Microscopic polyangiitis** (MPA)
- **Eosinophilic granulomatosis with polyangiitis** (EGPA, previously Churg–Strauss syndrome)

*Rheumatology Board Review*, First Edition. Edited by Karen Law and Aliza Lipson.
© 2014 John Wiley & Sons, Inc. Published 2014 by John Wiley & Sons, Inc.

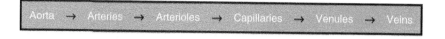

Aorta → Arteries → Arterioles → Capillaries → Venules → Veins

Large vessel vasculitis

- Age >50 → **Giant cell arteritis**
- Age <50 → **Takaysu arteritis**

Medium vessel vasculitis

- Necrotizing vasculitis, primarily in children, with associated mucocutaneous lymph node syndrome → **Kawasaki disease**
- Necrotizing vasculitis, primarily in adults, without mucocutaneous lymph node syndrome → **Polyarteritis nodosa**

Small vessel vasculitis

- Necrotizing vasculitis without immune deposits → <u>ANCA-associated vasculitis</u>
    - Eosinophilia, eosinophilic-predominant granulomatous disease, asthma → **EGPA**/Churg–Strauss
    - Neutrophilic-predominant granulomatous disease without asthma (may still have lung involvement) → **GPA**/Wegener's granulomatosis
    - No granulomatous disease → **Microscopic polyangiitis**
- Immune deposits present
    - IgA-containing immune complexes, primarily in venules → **IgA vasculitis**/Henoch–Schonlein purpura
    - Cryoglobulin deposits → **Cryoglobulinemic vasculitis**
    - Preceding or concomitant rheumatic disease (i.e. SLE, RA, etc.) → **Vasculitis secondary to rheumatic disease**
    - Recent new drug exposure with primarily palpable purpura and leukocytoclastic vasculitis, primarily in venules → **Hypersensitivity vasculitis**
    - Concomitant viral infection, i.e. hepatitis B, C, HIV, syphilis, malignancy, etc. → **Vasculitis secondary to infection or other probable etiology**

**Figure 13.1** Classification of vasculitis. (Source: Adapted from Jennette, J.C., Falk, R.J., Bacon, P.A. et al. (2013) 2012 Revised International Chapel Hill Consensus Conference Nomenclature of Vasculitides. *Arthritis and Rheumatism* 65(1): 1–11; and Fries, J.F., Hunder, G.G., Bloch, D.A., et al. (1990) The American College of Rheumatology 1990 criteria for the classification of vasculitis. *Arthritis and Rheumatism* 33(8): 1135–1136.)

## What are ANCAs?

• ANCAs are serologic markers for AAV, and are autoantibodies directed against granular and lysosomal components of neutrophils

• Fluorescent staining patterns are determined by indirect immunofluorescence and distinguish cytoplasmic ANCA (C-ANCA) staining patterns from perinuclear (P-ANCA) staining patterns

• Direct testing of target antigens such as **proteinase-3 (PR3)** and **myeloperoxidase (MPO)** is often performed after C-ANCA or P-ANCA is detected by indirect immunofluorescence

   ○ The target antigen of C-ANCA is PR3

   ○ The target antigen of P-ANCA is MPO

   ○ PR3-ANCA are the predominant ANCA type in GPA, while MPO-ANCA are the predominant ANCA type in MPA and EGPA, though overlapping or atypical ANCA expression can be seen

• ANCAs are hypothesized to have a pathogenic role in the tissue inflammation and vascular injury seen in AAV

   ○ In vitro studies have shown that proinflammatory cytokines stimulate neutrophils to express ANCA target antigens on their cell surfaces; these neutrophils, when exposed to ANCA, degranulate, releasing enzymes that may induce vasculitic lesions

   ○ Animal studies have shown that infusion of anti-MPO IgG induces small vessel vasculitis including glomerulonephritis and pulmonary capillaritis

   ○ Limited case studies have shown that transplacental transfer of anti-MPO ANCA can result in neonatal pulmonary-renal disease

---

**Keep in mind**

Data from the use of rituximab in AAV (discussed later in this chapter) may invalidate the pathogenic role of ANCAs in AAV, as the majority of patients with AAV treated with rituximab achieve disease remission but do not become ANCA negative.

---

• New data suggest a role for antibodies to **LAMP-2**, a lysosomal membrane protein, in the pathogenesis of AAV

   ○ LAMP-2 is expressed on the intracellular vesicles of neutrophils, especially those vesicles containing MPO and PR3

   ○ Scientists hypothesize that exposure to an infectious agent may induce autoantibodies to LAMP-2 via molecular mimicry, thereby inducing neutrophil activation and expression of disease

○ Although reports vary, the presence of autoantibodies to LAMP-2 has been reported in up to 90% of patients with AAV, with a rapid decline in antibody levels between disease flares

○ Additional studies are necessary to fully characterize the role of anti-LAMP-2 antibodies in AAV

## Treatment of AAV
### Conventional treatment of AAV
• For decades, corticosteroids with traditional immunosuppressants, such as cyclophosphamide, have been the foundation of induction therapy in AAV, followed by maintenance therapy with azathioprine or methotrexate

○ Cyclophosphamide may be given PO or IV

■ Rates of remission are comparable between the two dosing routes

■ Monthly IV cyclophosphamide is associated with a lower total cyclophosphamide dose and lower rates of leukopenia, but higher relapse rates

○ Both methotrexate and azathioprine are equivalent in maintaining remission after induction therapy

○ Mycophenolate mofetil has been shown in one study to be inferior to azathioprine in preventing relapse and therefore is not a first-line agent

• In patients with severe, active renal disease, limited data supports the addition of **plasma exchange** to traditional induction regimens of cyclophosphamide and corticosteroids; expert opinion also suggests a role for plasma exchange in the setting of pulmonary hemorrhage, though randomized studies have not been performed to establish superiority over standard care

• These regimens have improved survival, but are also associated with serious treatment-related adverse events; frequent relapses also add to substantial morbidity

○ Adverse events include:

■ Bone marrow suppression

■ Infertility

■ Malignancy, especially bladder cancer and lymphoma

■ Serious infection

■ Cystitis

### Rituximab in the treatment of AAV
• Two prospective, randomized controlled trials have examined rituximab for the treatment of AAV

- The RAVE trial established the non-inferiority of rituximab $375\,mg/m^2$ IV weekly for 4 weeks compared to oral cyclophosphamide in the induction therapy of AAV
  - Both groups received a similar regimen of pulse corticosteroids followed by a tapering corticosteroid regimen
  - Rituximab was found not to be inferior to cyclophosphamide ($p < 0.001$) at the primary endpoint on a standardized vasculitis activity scale (the Birmingham Vasculitis Activity Score)
  - There were no significant differences in adverse events between the two groups
  - Patients receiving treatment for relapsing disease had superior outcomes in the rituximab arm when compared to the cyclophosphamide arm
- The RITUXVAS trial, run concomitantly to the RAVE trial, also established the non-inferiority of rituximab weekly for 4 weeks with two IV cyclophosphamide doses compared to standard IV cyclophosphamide for 3–6 months followed by azathioprine in patients with AAV and severe renal disease
  - The rituximab group was found to be non-inferior to the cyclophosphamide group at the primary endpoint of remission at 12 months (76% of patients in the rituximab arm vs 82% in the cyclophosphamide arm, $p = ns$)
  - There were no significant differences in adverse events between the two groups
- The bottom line
  - Rituximab is a promising alternative to cyclophosphamide in induction therapy for moderately active AAV, and in 2011 became the first FDA-approved treatment for AAV
  - Rituximab may spare patients the toxicities customarily associated with cyclophosphamide, such as infertility, hemorrhagic cystitis, bone marrow suppression, and malignancy
  - Rituximab does appear to be superior to cyclophosphamide in patients with relapsed disease
  - The role of concomitant cyclophosphamide with rituximab (as in the RITUXVAS trial) needs to be further investigated
  - Maintenance therapy after rituximab has not yet been well established; in the RITUXVAS and RAVE studies, no maintenance therapy was given
  - While rituximab represents a paradigm-shifting development in the treatment of AAV, additional long-term studies are needed to address remaining questions, including:

- Rates of relapse after rituximab
- Long-term adverse effects
- Approach to re-treatment when a relapse occurs
- Role of rituximab or other agents in maintenance therapy
- Role of rituximab in severely ill patients with renal or respiratory failure

## ANCA-positive vasculitis mimics

New evidence from the study of ANCA as well as wider population testing for these antibodies has revealed that ANCA expression is not exclusive to the AAV and may be present in other disease states. Our understanding of these conditions continues to evolve.

- **CIMDL: cocaine-induced midline destructive lesions**
  - A condition causing necrosis and ulcerative erosions in the hard palate with nasal crusting and nasal septal perforation due to regular nasal cocaine use
  - Cocaine exposure and subsequent polyclonal B cell activation, similar to what occurs in allopurinol, PTU, or other drug exposure, induces falsely positive serum ANCA levels
  - Patients present with positive ANCA and elevated inflammatory markers
  - Given these manifestations, these patients can often be difficult to distinguish from limited GPA patients
  - The emerging role of **human neutrophil elastase** (HNE)
    - HNE is a serine protease with similar homology and gene localization to proteinase 3 (PR3)
    - HNE is common in CIMDL: in a series of 25 patients with CIMDL, 84% were HNE positive and 57% were PR3 positive
    - HNE is rare in autoimmune disease and vasculitis
      - → 0/174 patients with GPA or MPA were HNE positive
      - → 3/526 patients with other autoimmune diseases like ulcerative colitis or idiopathic thrombocytopenic purpura (ITP) were HNE positive

Therefore these characteristics enable HNE testing in patients with midline destructive lesions to be discriminatory between CIMDL and GPA. In these cases, PR3 testing alone may not be sufficient to distinguish the two diagnoses.

- Appropriate diagnosis between CIMDL and limited GPA is critical, as the treatment of CIMDL is withdrawal of the offending agent (cocaine), while treatment of GPA is with varying immunosuppressive medications
- **Levamisole-induced skin necrosis**
  - A newly described, increasingly reported condition
  - Levamisole is a veterinary antihelminth agent that is employed as a cocaine adulterant
  - Because it is cheap, widely available, and induces a euphoric-like feeling when inhaled, it is a common additive in up to 80% of cocaine in North America
  - Case reports show that toxicity from excess exposure to levamisole induces **skin necrosis**, primarily of the ears and extremities, **violaceous skin lesions, fever**, and **leukopenia**, in a condition that mimics vasculitis
  - Similar to CIMDL, patients may exhibit false-positive ANCA serologies
  - Confirmation of exposure to levamisole is tested through a urine screen, however metabolites to levamisole are only present within 24 hours of last use
  - Treatment of levamisole-induced skin necrosis involves withdrawal of the offending agent, with the majority of cases improving with this intervention alone
    - In severe cases with extensive skin necrosis, more rapid improvement has been reported with the use of systemic steroids

## Further reading

Bradford, M., Rosenberg, B., Moreno, J., Dumyati, G. (2010) Bilateral necrosis of earlobes and cheeks: another complication of cocaine contaminated with levamisole. *Annals of Internal Medicine* 152(11): 758–759.

Gomez-Puerta, J.A., Quintana, L.F., Stone, J.H., et al. (2012) B-cell depleting agents for ANCA vasculitides: a new therapeutic approach. *Autoimmunity Reviews* 11(9): 646–652.

Jayne, D.R., Gaskin, G., Rasmussen, N., et al. (2007) Randomized trial of plasma exchange or high-dosage methylprednisolone as adjunctive therapy for severe renal vasculitis. *Journal of the American Society of Nephrology* 18(7): 2180–2188.

Jones, R.B., Tervaert, J.W., Hauser, T., et al. (2010) Rituximab versus cyclophosphamide in ANCA-associated renal vasculitis. *New England Journal of Medicine* 363(3): 211–220.

Kain, R., Rees, A.J. (2013) What is the evidence for antibodies to LAMP-2 in the pathogenesis of ANCA associated small vessel vasculitis? *Current Opinion in Rheumatology* 25(1): 26–34.

Stone, J.H., Merkal, P.A., Spiera, R., et al. (2010) Rituximab versus cyclophosphamide for ANCA-associated vasculitis. *New England Journal of Medicine* 363(3): 221–232.

Trimarchi, M., Gregorini, G., Facchetti, F., et al. (2001) Cocaine-induced midline destructive lesions: clinical, radiographic, histopathologic, and serologic features and their differentiation from Wegener granulomatosis. *Medicine (Baltimore)* 80(6): 391–404.

Wiesner, O., Russell, K.A., Lee, A.S., et al. (2004) Antineutrophil cytoplasmic antibodies reacting with human neutrophil elastase as a diagnostic marker for cocaine-induced midline destructive lesions but not autoimmune vasculitis. *Arthritis and Rheumatism* 50(9): 2954–2965.

# Index

Figures are indicated in *italics;* tables are indicated in **bold**.

---

*Rheumatology Board Review,* First Edition. Edited by Karen Law and Aliza Lipson.
© 2014 John Wiley & Sons, Inc. Published 2014 by John Wiley & Sons, Inc.